BRIDGET HUNT

SIX PACK CHICK

ECADEMY PRESS

SIX PACK CHICK
Change Your Mind, Transform Your Body

First published in 2013 by Ecademy Press
48 St Vincent Drive, St Albans, Herts, AL1 5SJ
info@ecademy-press.com
www.ecademy-press.com

Printed and bound by Lightning Source in the UK and USA
Designed by Sophie Norman

Printed on acid-free paper from managed forests. This book is
printed on demand, so no copies will be remaindered or pulped.

ISBN 978-1-908746-22-1

A CIP catalogue record for this book is available from the
British Library.

This book is available online and all good bookstores.

Acknowledgments

I have so many people to acknowledge in writing this book – the list is endless, but here are the people who really have helped in my Six Pack Chick journey:

Dr John Briffa
Nathalie Eleni Bouziotas
Breda Gasjek
Dr Kim Jobst
John Hardy
Sylvie Walker
Michelle Zelli
Steve Bolton
Lindsay Jay
Mindy Gibbins-Klein
Darren Shirlaw
Michelle Warren
Daniel Priestley
Oliver Dudley
Mike Harris
Carlo Vagliasindi

All the chicks and chaps who have been clients and members of my support group – this book would not have happened without your determination, your amazing results and your love.

To Mum and Dad and Andy – thank you for always encouraging me to do what I believe in. Your love and support has got me to where I am today, and I am eternally grateful.

To Ollie – for your huge support and belief, in both me as a person, and for Six Pack Chick, the brand – I love you.

This book is really for everyone out there who obsesses about food and dieting. You are not alone.

Contents

Introduction

Are you sitting comfortably? Let's begin.

Before you start reading this book, I want you to go and make a cup of tea or coffee, and find a comfortable place to sit. Put your favourite slouchy clothes on, and raid the cupboards for any of your favourite comfort foods.

Turn the TV off and put on some nice background music (I like Michael Bublé **EVEN** though he's married now...sob).

Go and do it now. (Pause for five minutes.)
OK; comfortable? Then let's begin.

This book will change your life. It is a lifestyle book (not a diet) and encompasses mindset training and making exercise fun. You in turn will receive the following benefits:

1. **Health;**

2. **Vitality;**

3. **Self-belief.**

I know what it is like to be on a permanent diet. I know what it is like to be in a binge-and-then-guilt cycle. I spent years obsessing about my weight, about food and the pressure of trying to be thin. You may have picked up this book looking for answers as to why you are addicted to food, which will then help you find a way of eating that you can stick to, and therefore achieve long-term results. You have come to the right place.

Hatching the Chick

I don't know about you but I have tried just about every diet out there. I always used to start full of enthusiasm, and then I gave up after three days because it didn't fit in with my lifestyle.

I have researched many methods of losing body fat over the years and have gained great knowledge from some popular diets. Many of them have great properties, some of which are included in this book. It is mainly by trial and error with clients over the years that I have come up with a fat loss program that WORKS. It fits into every lifestyle. This book will give you all the tools you need to change your life. In a very short space of time, you will have more energy, have healthier skin, lose body fat, stop bloating and love your new self-image.

It appeals to everyone from teenagers to my mother (in her late sixties) and, with a little planning, you can easily and cheaply make it work for the rest of your life.

Now I hear you saying, "Yes Bridget, that's all great, but it is easy for you to say that – you **HAVE** a six-pack."

OK, so maybe I have now, but that was not always the case. I have been slim, slimmer, fat and fatter. I very rarely drink alcohol, but I have smoked, tried drugs and abused my body for years with refined carbohydrates. I know what it is to be obsessed with food. I know what it is like to eat a whole packet of biscuits instead of just the one. I know what emotional eating is and the horrible guilty feeling associated with it.

I have met hundreds of people over the years who go through a love/ hate relationship with food. Confused by all the diets, advice, quick fixes, media pressure, it is so easy to become obsessed and let your eating habits spiral out of control. I have often been awake long after everyone else is asleep, crying and silently giving myself a good telling off for the junk I have eaten that day – only to wake up in the morning and start the process all over again.

You are probably wondering what the benefits are? The following benefits are the results straight from my trial group and some of the personal benefits that I have found. They are divided into physical and psychological benefits.

Here is how Six Pack Chick works:

Necessary ingredients:
- A piece of string;
- An open mind;
- A cracking soundtrack to enjoy life.

You will get rid of the guilt associated with food.

You will join a thriving community on Facebook, people to support you, to bounce ideas off, to share recipes and to laugh with.

You will learn some key exercises that require 25 minutes per day, three days a week – with **NO GYM MEMBERSHIP**.

You will create a 'Bucket List' and have the confidence to get your dream job or take up a new hobby.

You will understand what **REAL** hunger is, and not the fake hunger you get when your body is craving more junk food.

You will have increased your energy levels, which will refresh your outlook on life.

You will be able to say no to foods you don't want to eat, and a big yes to the foods that you know will help.

You will be able to walk into a supermarket, without the temptation of having to buy junk food.

Before we start, I would like you to go and throw away your scales...
now. If you cannot throw them away (because a relative bought them
for you as a present), take the batteries out and find a use for the scales.

Suggestions:
- Cover it in a pretty cloth and stand a plant pot on it;
- Use it for when you have washed the kitchen floor and need to stand on something without getting your feet wet;
- Get a marker pen and write on it 'luggage scales', then get on the internet and book a holiday.

Get my drift?? I don't want you to use your scales, ever, ever, again.
They become an obsession and are not part of your new lifestyle.
Weight is irrelevant in this new lifestyle. What is more important to
you (honestly); to be a certain weight, or to be able to drop a few dress
sizes and fit into those skinny jeans that have been collecting dust in
your wardrobe (yes, I had a pair of those, too)?

What I want you to do is get some string, or pretty ribbon, or that
Christmas ribbon that you curl with a pair of scissors and use to wrap
presents.

1. **Get naked (check that you have closed the curtains);**
2. **Then tie the string/ribbon around your chest/bust and cut off when the two ends meet. Colour the end in felt tip or tie a label to it, marking chest/ bust;**
3. **Repeat with waist (the narrowest part);**
4. **Hips (the widest part);**

5. **The fattest bit of thigh (each one);**

6. **The fattest bit of upper arm;**

7. **When you are done, put all the labelled pieces of string in a plastic bag and keep in a safe place;**

8. **These are going to be your measurements from now on. No scales or tape measures; just plain, old-fashioned string or ribbon.**

Who can benefit from Six Pack Chick?

I have helped hundreds of clients with this method, and you will hear from those success stories later in the book (you can go and look at them now if you need some instant inspiration!). I get a lot of people coming to me for a quick fix. I can offer a quick fix; however, I turn that thought into a long-term strategy. I get clients saying they need to lose weight for their wedding, lose post-pregnancy weight, to get back on the magazine front cover after a period away from the media spotlight. Whatever their reason, I always say that it is 100% achievable, but first they need to change their relationship with food. You will find that this **DOES** give quick results and even better it's easy to follow the basic principles for the rest of your slim, confident life.

I also talk about various illnesses and the implications of diet on their health. I mention these specifically as these are the most prevalent amongst my clients.

Most of my clients are women between the ages of 30 to 50. That is not to say I exclusively work with that age range and gender. I work with obese teenagers and I have several clients in their 60s and 70s, who just want to get slim, and therefore they are full of energy and healthier as a result. We are in an era where everyone wants to feel good about themselves no matter what the number of years on their clock.

Here are a few key groups of people that can successfully follow Six Pack Chick; you may fit in one of these categories – if not then don't panic, as these are just examples:

Post-Pregnancy Chicks

The hormones are bouncing around, you are tired, sleep deprived and all you want to do is lose the post-pregnancy fat. You grab quick-fix food, and you are certainly having lots of sugar to try to boost your energy levels. If you are breast feeding, you are more likely to get rid of the baby bulge but not if you cram in vast quantities of chocolate, crisps, cake and sugar-laden lattes.

Not only can you lose the bulge effectively with Six Pack Chick, you will find that you will have MORE energy and not less by cutting out the sugar. Double bonus.

'Help I am getting married' Chicks

You have the wedding booked, the dress picked, the menu designed and now you are panicking because you simply want to look fabulous on the big day.

If you want to have a flat stomach, beautiful skin and glossy hair, then Six Pack Chick is for you. I have successfully used this method on over 100 brides to be. Not only do they look fabulous on their wedding day, but also they get some great bikini shots on their honeymoon!

Menopause Chicks (this is a big one)

You have always stayed the same size – give or take a few belt notches – and then menopause comes and bang...the waistline increases, bingo wings arrive and no matter what you do you can't seem to shift it.

Why does this happen?

Oestrogen: Oestrogen is the female sex hormone that is responsible for causing monthly ovulation. During female menopause, your oestrogen levels decline rapidly, causing your body to stop ovulating.

However, oestrogen also plays a major role in menopausal weight gain. As your ovaries produce less oestrogen, your body looks for other places for its oestrogen. Fat cells in your body can produce oestrogen, so your body works harder to convert calories into fat to increase oestrogen levels. Unfortunately for you, fat cells do not burn calories the way muscle cells do, which causes you to pack on the unwanted pounds.

Progesterone: During menopause, progesterone levels will also decrease. Like oestrogen, lower levels of this hormone can be responsible for many of the symptoms of menopause and that includes weight gain, or at least the appearance of it. Water retention and menopause often go hand in hand since water weight and bloating are caused by decreased progesterone levels. Though this does not actually result in weight gain, your clothes will probably feel a bit tighter and you may feel heavier. Water retention and bloating usually disappear within a few months.

Androgens: These hormones are responsible for sending your new weight directly to your middle section. In fact, weight gain during menopausal years is affectionately known as 'middle-aged spread' because of the rapid mid-section growth. Often, one of the first signs of menopause is an increase of androgen in your body, which causes you to gain weight around your abdominals instead of around your lower half.

Testosterone: Testosterone helps your body to create lean muscle mass out of the calories that you take in. Muscle cells burn more calories than fat cells, increasing your metabolism. In natural menopause, levels of testosterone drop, resulting in the loss of this muscle. Unfortunately, this means a lower metabolism. The lower your metabolism, the slower your body burns calories.

Other factors involved in weight gain during menopause

Insulin Resistance: Insulin resistance can occur during your menopausal years. This is when your body mistakenly turns every calorie you take in into fat. Most women follow a low-fat, high-carbohydrate diet. After time, processed and refined foods can make your body resistant to insulin produced in the bloodstream. This is often a cause of weight gain after the age of 40.

Stress: Stress is also a contributing factor in weight gain in menopause. Stress hormones can prevent weight loss as they signal to your body to go into a storage mode. This is referred to as the 'famine effect'. Your body, thinking it won't get food again for a long time, stores every calorie it takes in, causing weight gain.

I have a lot of menopause chicks, they find that everything improves – the sweats, skin, hair, energy levels and the waist becomes smaller and smaller. In fact, some of the greatest results that I get can be from this group of women.

You **CAN** get more fabulous as you get older!

Acne Chicks

Many of you reading this will know exactly what I mean when I say that acne, as an adult, is so frustrating. You go through puberty and spend half of it in a high street pharmacy trying out the latest acne creams only to ditch them when you are nineteen or so, thinking that was the end of it..Not in my case. I started getting full on spots in my 20s and tried almost everything to get rid of them. I didn't go quite as far as a paper bag, but almost...

Doctors have been saying for years that glucose does not lead to pimples. Latest research indicates they may be wrong. A study looked into whether Glycaemic Index (GI) has effect on pimples. Glycaemic Index is the measurement to show how quickly a carbohydrate (glucose is a carbohydrate) makes its way into the bloodstream. The higher the GI of a food, the faster the sugar is absorbed. The study, reported at the Journal of the American Academy of Dermatology, compared the impact of normal (higher GI) diet plan to a low GI eating habits. The findings? Individuals on the low GI diet plan had far fewer pimples than the control group eating the high GI diet plan.

Conclusion: *glucose and other high Glycaemic Index foods have an effect on acne breakouts.*

By way of summarising the study and translating from medical jargon into plain English, you do not need to get a PhD just to understand it.

Dr Cordain states that fluctuations in blood sugar level cause acne by:
- Increasing sebum production;
- Causing skin cells to regenerate faster;
- Causing dead skin cells to stick together.

Faster regeneration of skin cells means that more dead skin cells have to be pushed through skin pores. (By the way, it also means faster aging of skin.) When dead skin cells stick together, they have to be pushed through skin pores in big lumps instead of single skin cells. It is like diverting heavy truck traffic through a narrow village road: that can only mean traffic jams.

Throw in a good measure of sticky sebum and it can only lead to one thing: clogged skin pores and acne.

Polycystic Ovary Syndrome (PCOS) Chicks

For years, I took the contraceptive pill Dianette. It was prescribed to me by my GP, who for no other reason, decided that I would, 'get on well with it'. Several GPs and two decades later, I decided to stop taking it, as I had read horror stories about it, and I wanted to think about having children. After being pill-free for six months with no menstrual cycle, I then decided to investigate. To my complete shock it was discovered that I had Polycystic Ovary Syndrome.

I had acne, hair loss, hair gain (where you don't want it), weight gain around my middle amongst other symptoms. If I wanted to get pregnant I would just have to get on with it, so I was told (nice advice), and that if I didn't, I could go back on the pill to help the symptoms (more great advice).

Deciding to take matters into my own hands, I set about fine-tuning the SPC method to see if it helped my symptoms.

Avoiding the daily spikes in blood sugar by designing a way of eating that keeps it stable has really helped my PCOS symptoms and now my menstrual cycle is completely back to normal.

Dr John Briffa, GP and nutritionist and author of The Waist Disposal, talks about Polycystic Ovary Syndrome in his excellent blog:

"Polycystic ovarian syndrome (PCOS) is a condition characterised by multiple cysts in the ovaries, but also other symptoms such as hirsutism (abnormal hairiness) and acne that may result from higher than normal levels of androgens ('male' hormones) in the female body. I wrote about this condition back in 2003, where I made the point that the best diet, generally speaking, was one based on low Glycaemic

Index (low GI) foods – i.e. foods that release sugar relatively slowly into the bloodstream.

One of the rationales here is that women with PCOS tend to be insulin resistant. In other words, their insulin tends not to work so well. The chief function of insulin is to reduce blood sugar levels. Therefore, if insulin isn't working too well, it makes sense to avoid eating foods that cause spikes in blood sugar. Furthermore, there is an idea that higher levels of insulin (common in insulin resistance) can stimulate androgen release. At the time, the idea of eating a low-GI diet was based on common sense and first principles. Recently, though, a group of scientists decided to test the merits of low-GI eating in the real world. [1]

96 women started the study, and were assigned to either a low-GI diet or a 'healthy' diet. In both diets, half of the calories were made up from carbohydrate. For each diet, calories contributed by protein and fat were the same, too (23 and 27 per cent), respectively. The overall GIs of the two diets were 40 and 59 respectively. The study lasted for 12 months.

A number of measures were taken, as part of the study including body composition, sex hormone levels, and blood sugar control (as assessed with an oral glucose tolerance test).

Compared to the group eating the standard diet, those eating the lower-GI diet saw significant improvement in the results of the glucose tolerance test, which would point to improved blood sugar control and insulin action.

In addition, 95 per cent of women saw improvement in the regularity of their menstrual cycle, compared to 63 per cent of the other group.

Overall, the lower-GI group did better, in other words.

This study provides some objective evidence that a low-GI diet has merit for women with PCOS. However, my advice for women with PCOS looking to improve their condition through diet is not to eat a low-GI diet, but to eat a low-carbohydrate one. The thing is; it is possible to eat a low-GI diet and still eat a lot of carbohydrates. In essence, the less carbohydrates someone eats, the less insulin they secrete and, in theory at least, the better the result."

I'm in agreement with Dr Briffa, that although low-GI diets go some way towards helping PCOS patients, they don't go far enough. Needing to know the Glycaemic Index of foods is also a pain – who wants to carry around lists of the GI score of individual foods in their handbag? Not me! I would rather leave the space for protein powder and SPC snacks on the go!

If you have been diagnosed with PCOS, then do not despair! Come and give SPC a try and see your symptoms improve.

Diseases and the implications of diet

As previously mentioned, in this section I will be talking about the implications of diet on specific illnesses. Whilst you may not be a sufferer, perhaps you have a friend or family member who is, and therefore you can go a long way in helping them by recommending Six Pack Chick.

Insulin resistance

Insulin resistance is an inability of some of the cells of the body to respond to insulin. It is the beginning of the body not dealing well with sugar (and remember that all carbohydrate breaks down into sugar in our bodies). One of insulin's main jobs is to get certain body cells to 'open up' to take in glucose (to store the glucose as fat). Insulin resistance happens when the cells do not open the door when insulin comes knocking. When this happens, the body puts out more insulin to stabilise blood glucose (and so the cells can use the glucose). Over time, this results in a condition called 'hyperinsulinemia' or too much insulin in the blood. Hyperinsulinemia causes other problems, including making it more difficult for the body to use fat for energy.

What causes insulin resistance?

Scientists do not know the whole story, but certainly genetics play a big part. Some people are actually born insulin-resistant. Lack of physical activity causes the cells to be less responsive to insulin. Most experts agree that obesity leads to more insulin resistance. However, it almost certainly works the other way around: insulin resistance promotes weight gain. Therefore, a vicious cycle can be set up with insulin resistance promoting weight gain, which promotes more insulin resistance.

What problems does insulin resistance cause?

Besides general weight gain, insulin resistance is associated with abdominal obesity, high blood pressure, high triglycerides, and low HDL ('good cholesterol'). These conditions are part of a constellation of problems called metabolic syndrome (also called insulin resistance syndrome). Because this group of symptoms occurs together, it is hard to know what causes what, but metabolic syndrome is a risk factor for heart disease and Type 2 diabetes.

Obesity

Obesity is all over the headlines; both in the UK and in the USA. It is currently on the rise, and requests for bariatric surgery and 'stomach stapling' are gathering pace at a daily rate.

I understand that a lot of clinically obese patients are fed up, depressed and feel that there is no alternative. I would love to help every one of the millions of obese patients out there. If they could come and join the SPC group and have the amazing support it offers, then we could go a long way in helping them. If you feel that you fit into the obese category then there is good news for you! I have successfully helped hundreds of obese patients shift considerable body fat and many of them are going on to help other people. The Six Pack Chick method is simple, fun and, with a bit of planning, very, very, easy to follow and with great results.

I want to have whole families doing it, friends and neighbours helping each other out and spreading the word that there IS a solution and they will get much needed personal support.

Candida

Candida is controversial. The medical profession denies its existence, except in very limited cases, making it very difficult (probably impossible) to get a medical diagnosis of candida, even when an overgrowth has been confirmed by a laboratory test. Despite this situation, public awareness of candida has continued to grow, helped no doubt by the long list of celebrities who, quite unperturbed by its lack of medical status, assert that they have had it.

Candida is the popular term for candidiasis (candida overgrowth) – a condition first identified by American physicians in the 1970s. Moderate amounts of candida live quite happily inside us, but when they are given free permission to grow unchecked, e.g. by wiping out the surrounding bacteria with broad-spectrum antibiotics, candida can change into its fungal form and spore through the intestinal wall into the rest of the body. However, once through, it wreaks havoc around the body producing a multitude of symptoms.

Common symptoms of candida
There are too many symptoms to list here. A minority of suffers have numerous symptoms; the vast majority have thrush + a few others; not every sufferer has thrush.

Group 1: The damage to the intestinal wall allows undesirable toxins to permeate into the bloodstream. This condition called 'leaky gut syndrome' often leads to:
- food allergies;
- foggy brain;
- migraines;
- muscle aches.

Group 2: Once through to the rest of the body, candida has the ability to disrupt the endocrine system (hormone secreting glands) causing symptoms such as:
- thrush;

- fungal infections of the nails/skin e.g. athlete's foot;
- cystitis;
- weight gain or weight loss;
- PMS;
- menstrual irregularities;
- joint pains;
- ear infections;
- asthma;
- chronic tiredness;
- hay fever;
- allergies;
- sinusitis;
- sensitivity to perfume, tobacco smoke and petrol.

Group 3: Symptoms in the intestines include:
- bloating;
- diarrhoea and/or constipation;
- flatulence;
- itchy anus.

In addition, candida involvement has been implicated in some cases of other illnesses, e.g. ME/chronic fatigue, endometriosis.

Before you all get anxious and wonder if you have it, I have with permission from Dr Crooks, given you a questionnaire towards the back of the book, which you can use to indicate whether you may have it and I have also given you details of a lab that I use to test for it properly.

You can use the spit test, too; it costs nothing and is quite indicative: The night before, leave a glass of water beside your bed. Immediately upon waking in the morning, before you do anything, spit into a glass of water. If your spit remains floating in a nice, cohesive 'blob', you are probably pretty much candida-free.

If after a few seconds, the spit begins to develop long strand-like tendrils that dissolve down into the water, or if your spit spreads out over the surface of the water, you probably have a candida condition. You can also then do the questionnaire towards the back of the book. The Six Pack Chick method works very well for candida sufferers. However, you will not be able to do the treat day for six to nine weeks. This will give you time to help the candida overgrowth to die off. Then you can start reintroducing fruit on your treat day, step-by-step.

Cancer
Sugar feeds cancer
The simple concept that 'sugar feeds cancer' is often overlooked as part of a comprehensive support plan for cancer sufferers. Out of the four million+ cancer patients being treated in the US today, few are offered specific advice or guidelines for using optimum nutrition, beyond being told to, 'just eat good foods'. Most cancer sufferers lack knowledge of what an optimal nutritional program is or how to implement it.

Many cancer sufferers could have a major improvement in the outcome of their disease if its preferred fuel, glucose, was controlled. Eliminating refined sugar and adopting an optimal wholefoods diet, combined with top quality nutritional supplements and exercise, may be critical components in recovering from cancer.

Glucose: the fuel of cancer cells
Dr Otto Warburg, Ph.D., a 1931 Nobel Laureate in medicine, first

discovered that cancer cells have a different energy metabolism compared to healthy cells. He found that malignant tumours frequently exhibit an increase in anaerobic ('without air') glycolysis – an abnormal process whereby glucose is used as a primary fuel by cancer cells, which generates large amounts of lactic acid as a by-product. [2]

In contrast, normal cells predominantly undergo aerobic ('with air') cellular metabolism. In cancer, the large increase in lactic acid generated by the cancer cells must be transported to the liver for metabolism and clearance. The lactic acid creates a lower, more acidic pH in cancerous tissues, as well as overall physical fatigue from liver stress due to overworking to try to clear the lactic acid buildup. [3/4] Consequently, larger tumours tend to have a more acidic pH. [5] The goal is to return the body to aerobic metabolism as quickly as possible and to achieve an alkaline tissue pH (6.4–7.0). An alkaline environment is an unfavourable environment for cancer growth. Since the cancer cell's metabolism, anaerobic glycolysis, is very inefficient, extracting only about 5% of the available energy in the food supply and from the body's own calorie stores, the cancer, in effect, is 'wasting' energy, so the cancer sufferer eventually becomes tired and undernourished. This vicious cycle increases body wasting – often in a downward spiral until death. [6] This is one reason why almost 40% of cancer sufferers die from malnutrition (called cachexia or 'wasting away'). [7]

Do glucose IVs feed cancer?
In hospitals, the total parenteral (TPN) solution typically given to cancer patients intravenously provides 70% of the calories going into the bloodstream in the form of glucose. These high-glucose solutions for cachectic cancer patients may be a poor choice of IV nutrition and may, in effect, be effectively feeding the tumour. A more nutritionally

balanced IV solution with low glucose levels, in addition to a broad spectrum of nutrients such as amino acids, vitamins, minerals, lipids and co-factors, may be a much better choice and allow the patient to build strength without feeding the tumor. [8]

The best ways to regulate blood-glucose levels in cancer sufferers may be the following:

1. **an optimal wholefoods diet;**

2. **top quality nutritional supplements with a broad spectrum of anti-infective, immune-supportive phytonutrients;**

3. **regular exercise and sunlight;**

4. **gradual weight loss (if overweight) and,**

5. **stress reduction. Professional nutritional guidance is crucial for cancer victims. The goal of nutrition therapy is not to eliminate all carbohydrates from the diet, but to eliminate all refined carbohydrates and thus, control blood glucose within a narrow range to help starve the cancer and also bolster immune function.**

Blood sugar standards

'Sugar' is a generic term used to identify simple and complex carbohydrates, which includes monosaccharides such as fructose, glucose and Galactose, and disaccharides such as maltose and sucrose (white table sugar). The standards for blood sugar levels are: a) less than 110 mg/dL is considered normal; b) 111 to 125 mg/dL is considered to be impaired glucose tolerance, and c) 26 mg glucose/dL blood or greater is considered to be diabetic (1997 American Diabetes Association blood-glucose standards).

Excess blood sugar and degeneration

The diet of our ancestors which consisted of vegetables, lean meat, whole grains, nuts, seeds and fruits, is estimated to have promoted healthy blood glucose levels between 60 and 90 mg/dL. [9] Today's typical diet, high in refined sugar, is promoting abnormally high blood sugar levels and unprecedented unhealthy effects in blood-sugar metabolism. Excess blood glucose can initiate yeast overgrowth, blood vessel deterioration, diabetes, heart disease, increased rate of infections and many other adverse health conditions. [10]

Blood sugar and breast cancer

A mouse-model of human breast cancer demonstrated that tumours are sensitive to blood glucose levels. Mice were injected with an aggressive strain of breast cancer, and then fed diets to induce one of the following: high blood sugar (hyperglycaemia), normal blood sugar, or low blood sugar (hypoglycaemia). The findings showed that the lower the blood glucose, the greater the survival rate. [11/12] This suggests that reducing refined sugar intake is a key factor in slowing breast tumour growth.

A large-scale epidemiological study of 21 modern countries that tracks morbidity and mortality (Europe, North America, Japan and others) revealed that sugar intake is a strong risk factor that contributes to higher breast cancer rates, particularly in older women. [13]

Blood sugar and immune cell activity

In an immune cell study, ten healthy people were assessed for fasting, blood-glucose levels and the phagocytic index of neutrophils, which measures the ability of immune cells to destroy invaders such as cancer. Eating 100 grams of carbohydrates from glucose, sucrose, honey and orange juice all significantly decreased the capacity of neutrophils to engulf bacteria. Starch did not have this effect. [14]

In a four-year research study at the National Institute of Public Health and Environmental Protection in the Netherlands, 111 cancer patients (with cancer of the biliary tract) were compared with 480 controls. Cancer risk associated with the intake of sugars, independent of other energy sources, more than doubled for the cancer patients. [15]

The medical establishment may be missing the connection between sugar and its role in tumorigenesis. The PET scan, a million-dollar positive emission tomography device, is regarded as one of the ultimate cancer-detection tools. PET scans use radioactively-labelled glucose to detect sugar-hungry tumour cells. The more glucose that is detected at a site, the worse the tumour is becoming. PET scans are used to plot the progress of cancerous tumours and to assess whether present protocols are effective. [16]

Kick the sugar out

In Europe, the 'sugar feeds cancer' concept is well known. Glucose has an irrefutable role in encouraging the growth and metastasis of cancer. Based on research and the cancer-sugar connection, the best dietary recommendation for those with cancer may be a wholefoods, organic diet. This will include more fresh, organic vegetables, but less sweet fruit (such as bananas, figs, dates, etc.), as well as eliminating all refined sugars, (such as fructose, sucrose, sorbitol, maltodextrin, etc.) including hidden refined sugars (found in foods not normally associated with containing sugar such as soups, breads, ketchup, etc.). This carefully planned regime may be an enormous help in regulating blood glucose and hence, improving immunity while selectively starving cancer cells.

Counting calories is futile and other diet mistakes I have made

I have tried every diet out there; I have eaten nothing but grapefruits for a week, and I have tried food combining (or not combining it should be called). Here are a few of the diets I have tried and why they did not work:

Cabbage soup diet

OK, this is preparing foul-smelling soup that you are required to drink large quantities of every day. My apartment smelt of rotting cabbages every time I stepped in through the front door and it gave me terrible flatulence. I got sick of the soup after three days and promptly ended it. I celebrated the end by bingeing on chocolate hob-nobs.

Counting calories

I was a master at counting calories; it became an obsession. At first, I carried a calculator everywhere with me, which made me look like an accountant. That space in my handbag is put to better use with a bigger make-up bag.

Counting calories takes ages out of your day, precious time wasted that could be put to better use by way of shoe-shopping or cooking something decent. It is dull and what on earth do you do if you get invited to dinner at a friend's house? "Er, excuse me, this is going to sound really strange, but do you know how many calories are in that big wedge of potato dauphinoise you just gave me?" Hmmmm. Not the best way to keep your friends.

The obsession just fuels internal unhappiness when you are shopping in the supermarket and you realise that what you really want to eat has too many calories. You then do a juggling act with what is in your basket and put something back to 'lessen' the calorific load for the day. Counting calories made me so unhappy and so stressed at the thought of going food shopping that it was no longer a pleasure – it was a chore.

Food combining

When I read some of the research into food combining; I decided to give it a go. I liked the sound of the idea that it was difficult for the body to digest both proteins and carbohydrates at the same time, so I started it off with gusto!

Whilst I felt a bit better, I really struggled when I was invited to friends' houses for dinner. These were the pre-Atkins days, when it was incomprehensible that you would eat just protein and vegetables for dinner and I got scuppered so many times because there, sitting in front of me in all its glory, was a delicious lasagne. If you have ever tried to pick bits of meat out of a lasagne you will know what I mean when I say it takes two hours to dissect with a fork and it looks like you have some crazy food problem. Not cool.

Another problem for me was that I did not understand that refined carbohydrates made me feel bad, so I would happily gorge myself on a dinner of pasta and tomato sauce only to feel **REALLY** hungry an hour later, bloated and irritable.

There are lots of diets out there that work really well for some people. I try not to slam any diet; if it works for someone, then great! One problem that I have with the word 'diets' though, is that people tend to get obsessed with them. They think of them as a quick fix rather than a long-term way of eating. If you have ever dieted then you know exactly what I mean by that. You start with great enthusiasm at the beginning and throw yourself into it only to sabotage after one, seven or 30 days when you cannot stick to it. Many of my dietary beliefs, used with Six Pack Chick, draw from some really successful methods out there. I have found the best principles, applied scientific research and created a sustainable, long-term program that gives great results.

Emotional eating

This is quite a big chapter (apologies but it is essential reading). From my own personal experience, emotional eating has been a big reason for my fluctuating body fat over the years. It also affects nine out of ten of all my female patients.

Here are a few questions that you may want to answer straight away or think about for a while before you keep reading. Even if you do not feel that you are an emotional eater, you may have a family member or friend who is and you can help them with the information in this book.

1.   **Do you spend a lot of your day thinking about food?**

2.   **Do you eat when you are not hungry?**

3.   **Do you ever go on eating binges for no apparent reason?**

4.   **Do you have feelings of guilt and remorse after binging on food?**

5.   **Do you have a sensible diet in front of others, and then go home and 'pig out' on rubbish?**

6.   **Do you get strong cravings to eat at times other than mealtimes?**

7.   **Do you overeat or binge when you are stressed or depressed?**

8.   **Does the way you respond to food worry your family and friends?**

I understand that many of these questions may make you feel uncomfortable and perhaps already have you reaching for the biscuit tin. Stay strong and keep reading, as we are going to put a stop to that feeling!

Emotional eating; why sometimes you cannot say **NO**.
I believe that emotional overeating is just like drug or alcohol abuse and even gambling. It is easy to compare it to drug abuse – over exposure to the feeling of elation that the user has after taking in the drug conditions the body to crave it time and time again. After a while, this repeated pattern leads to a feeling that they have lost control, they no longer feel satisfied with the specific 'dose' they were taking and they start to obsess about where their next fix is coming from. The same can be said for people addicted to alcohol, to prescription painkillers and even those addicted to sex.

Food can be just as addictive. Sugar, fat and salt all carry their own feelings of elation when consumed and, when they are all eaten together, it can be impossible to stop once started.

Most women I talk to experience food cravings and overeating at various stages in their life. I used to think it was just a PMT thing – you know, a couple of days before when not only do you cry at the smallest things, you would rugby tackle a complete stranger to the floor if they were holding a big bar of chocolate and all the shops were shut.

Whether it's having an overwhelming urge to eat something sweet after dinner or opening a packet of biscuits mid afternoon to have 'just the one' with a cup of tea (and then eating five or six), then craving sugar can be a powerful urge. Unfortunately, the truth is that once we start to include sugar in our daily routine, it becomes more and more difficult to stop.

So why can't we just say No?

As humans we have evolved to appreciate the instant energy sugar provides us, but food is a highly emotional topic, especially when it comes to sweets. We often associate sweet foods with love and acceptance. Scientists have looked at our brain chemistry to understand how food can directly affect our 'feel-good' chemicals and this is where dopamine comes in.

Research on the brain indicates that addiction is about powerful memories and recovery is a slow process in which the influence of those memories is diminished. Both addictive drugs and highly pleasurable or intense experiences (such as a life or death thrill, a crime, or an orgasm) trigger the release of the brain chemical dopamine, which in turn creates a reward circuit in the brain. This circuit registers that intense experience as 'important' and creates lasting memories of it as a pleasurable experience. Dopamine changes the brain on a cellular level, commanding the brain to 'do it again', which heightens the possibility of relapse even long after the behaviour (or drug) has stopped. Dopamine also helps to explain why sugar can be just as addictive as drugs.

(Now for a bit of science!)

Gene Jack-Wang, a physician at Brookhaven Lab and the Mount Sinai School of Medicine in America, conducted a trial and the results were published online on February 24, 2011. In the journal Obesity, his findings suggest that the dopamine spike may play a role in triggering compulsive overeating:

"These results identify dopamine neurotransmission, which primes the brain to seek reward, as being of relevance to the neurobiology of binge eating disorder."

Previous studies conducted by Wang's team have identified a similar dopamine spike in drug-addicted individuals when they were shown images of people taking drugs, as well as other neurochemical similarities between drug addiction and obesity, including a role for dopamine in triggering desire for drugs and/or food.

"In earlier studies of normal-weight healthy people who had been food-deprived for 16 hours, we found that dopamine releases were significantly correlated with self-reports of hunger and desire for food. These results provided evidence of a conditioned-cue response to food," Wang said.

Thanks dopamine, that's really helpful!

Sadly, we have been told for far too long that indulging in sweets is connected with a lack of self-will or some other character flaw. This is complete rubbish; I have a very strong will in lots of areas in my life but not where sugar is involved. Craving sugar is not simply about willpower, nor is it simply about emotions. There may be several underlying physiological causes feeding your desire for sugar; we now know that dopamine is one, but what else is behind it?

Why does sugar feel so good?
There are so many contributions to the positive feelings we associate with sugar. For many of us, the smell of home-made brownies or a cake fresh out of the oven reminds us of our childhoods, evoking fond memories of past holidays, birthdays, or special occasions. Others remember being rewarded with sweets or other sugar-filled treats when they did something 'good', like passed an exam or tidied their room.

These positive associations are ingrained in our brains from a very early age. Years ago, at the start of my health problems, I went to see a nutritionist and he advised that I cut sugar out of my diet for a week. I remember the feeling of panic very clearly; it was as if someone was suggesting I did not ever see my best friend again, like I was being punished for doing something wrong. Some clients respond in the same way when I tell them; the instant reaction when someone tells you that you can't have something is to both cry for it **AND** eat as much of it as possible before you give it up. (I did stop at the shop after that consultation years ago and eat a big bag of Maltesers.)

The more I have delved into this sugar problem over the years, the more it makes sense. Now let's talk about serotonin.

Serotonin is the feel-good hormone, amongst other things. It is a neurotransmitter and neurotransmitters work by sending messages from the nervous system to the rest of the body; serotonin levels are what several antidepressants manipulate to improve mood and anxiety.

Made from the essential amino acid, tryptophan, serotonin's roots are in protein. So what does sugar have to do with it? The reason sugar can lead to increased serotonin in the brain has to do with insulin. I'll explain this in more detail below, but the bottom line is that we need insulin to help tryptophan get into the brain so it can produce serotonin. In addition, sugar – or any carbohydrate for that matter – causes us to release insulin. Refined carbohydrates, such as sugar, white bread, pasta and white rice, lead to a more intense insulin surge than complex carbohydrates like vegetables.

Another neurotransmitter that I want to talk about is beta-endorphin. We release this when eating sweets or refined carbohydrates. This is the neurotransmitter typically associated with a 'runner's high' because it acts as a natural painkiller, produces a sense of well-being, increases self-esteem, and settles anxiety. Our brains naturally release beta-endorphin when we are in any kind of physical pain – and when we eat sugar.

It's no wonder sugar feels so good! Physiologically, sugar 'feeds' our brains with three neurotransmitters that send positive messages to the rest of the body. The problem is that the high we experience after a big fat piece of chocolate cake, a bowl of special fried rice, or a bag of Maltesers, does not last very long, and eating these foods, especially without combining them with some protein, can set us up for cyclical cravings. You just want to eat more and more of it.

Is sugar addictive?

So many people ask me whether sugar is addictive; the true answer differs depending on the individual. Sugar certainly can be addictive (especially in my case), but it is more of a problem for some people than others, because we all have different levels of these neurotransmitters and receptors in our brains.

These levels vary and change over time depending upon our genetics and lifestyle – what we eat, drink and feel; where we are hormonally; whether we exercise; how well we sleep; and so on. Some practitioners believe that a proportion of the population is 'sugar-sensitive'. These individuals may be operating with naturally lower levels of serotonin and beta-endorphin, leaving them more vulnerable to sugar cravings. Let's think about it as supply and demand; any time the body is running low on a neurotransmitter, the brain tries to catch up by opening up more receptors for this neurotransmitter, essentially to increase the odds of a connection. When there is less of something floating around there is more of a need for it. With so many open receptors, if a sugar-sensitive person does have sugar, alcohol, or anything that causes a release of serotonin or beta-endorphin, it intensifies the resulting sugar 'high'. This in turn can lead to more cravings.

If you try to think about a situation where your sugar consumption got out of control, you will understand what I mean. I remember feeling very anxious about attending a hospital appointment. I craved sugar like you wouldn't believe and, once I started, I couldn't stop. After the appointment, my blood sugar had come crashing down and I ate more sugar, also wanting to reward myself for having got through the traumatic experience. I then had a migraine for three days; a combination of all the sugar and the stress of what I had been through...double whammy.

You may find, when starting Six Pack Chick, that you suffer withdrawal symptoms when you stop eating sugar. This makes sense because when we are eating large amounts of sugar at regular intervals, the brain becomes accustomed to frequent beta-endorphin bursts and, when we take them away, it naturally wants more. This, like withdrawal from a caffeine habit or drug addiction, can lead to headaches, shakiness, nausea, fatigue, and even depression.

Your body needs carbohydrates
It may be tempting for women who feel they have a problem with sugar to cut out all carbohydrates. However, an all-or-nothing approach just isn't healthy – it takes all four food groups to regulate insulin and quell sugar cravings. Here is an explanation for why.

Whenever we eat foods that contain complex carbohydrates, our bodies convert them into a simple sugar known as glucose. Glucose is the main source of fuel for our cells. The brain in particular cannot use any other source of energy (like fat or protein) aside from glucose, so it is essential to eat carbohydrates.

As I mentioned earlier, carbohydrates are also important in helping tryptophan get into the brain to be converted to serotonin. When we eat food containing protein, the body breaks it down into subcomponent amino acids – one of which is tryptophan.

The tryptophan molecule is relatively small compared to other amino acids. Those larger amino acids can block tryptophan's path across the tightly regulated barrier between the blood and the brain. When carbohydrates are consumed and insulin is released, insulin pairs up with larger amino acids to help build muscle, leaving tryptophan a clearer path to cross into the brain. Moreover, there are important micronutrients, such as vitamin C, the B vitamins, and zinc (see box at right), that can help with the conversion from tryptophan to serotonin.

What is interesting is that Mother Nature did not provide our bodies with the information to distinguish between man-made sugars and natural sugars. Instead, this information is available to us in everything else that surrounds natural sugars – in the antioxidant-rich skins of grapes and apples, for example, or the fibre and protein-rich germ of whole grains.

Therefore, eating any kind of sweet or refined carbohydrate will satisfy the brain and increase serotonin – but it won't trigger the signals that tell our brain that we have had enough, that we are now fully sated. The more refined a food is, the more it has been stripped of these natural, information-rich fibres, fats, proteins, vitamins and antioxidants.

The carbohydrates in white flours, white rice, white sugar and the majority of pastas and breakfast cereals are all highly refined. Therefore, it takes less time for the body to break them down, leading to a quicker response all round. This may sound good, but in the long run, quick spikes in insulin and glucose can damage your metabolism and lead to insulin resistance and more cravings. There are so many delicious complex carbohydrates to choose from that will gently increase blood sugar and insulin. Vegetables and pulses are excellent choices.

Possible causes for sugar cravings

As I mentioned earlier, sugar cravings often have many facets. Because eating is so intimately connected with our biochemistry and our emotions, we 'digest' sugar on many levels. You may notice there's a pattern to when you crave sugar – for so many of my patients it is cyclical, occurring nightly after a stressful day at work, monthly just before their periods, or seasonally, when the days grow short. For others, sugar binges may be connected to the kinds of foods they have already eaten that day, or with a daily ritual. Here are some of the common causes for sugar cravings I see at the clinic:

Hormonal fluctuations: Just before menstruation, when oestrogen is low and progesterone is on its way down, beta-endorphin levels are at their lowest. These cyclical hormonal and neurotransmitter fluctuations may explain why many women who experience PMS also have cravings – and the accompanying serotonin/ endorphin bursts that high-sugar foods can provide.

Stress: Any stressful situation can lead to less than optimal eating habits. Stress itself increases cortisol levels, which initially dampen hunger. Once the stress has abated, our hormones of hunger ramp up – "Refuel!" the body cries. This can lead many women with stressful jobs and lifestyles to a pattern of night-time cravings, over-eating, and unwanted weight gain. Over time, chronic stress can lead to adrenal fatigue, eventually resulting in extreme exhaustion. So many women I see have reached a state of adrenal fatigue and find the only way to get through the day is by drinking lots of caffeine and consuming sugar for quick energy bursts. However, this only sets them up for further cravings and more energy depletion. There are many simple ways to support your adrenal health by what and how you eat.

Insulin resistance: When you are resistant to insulin (which can happen as a result of a long-term diet high in refined carbohydrates and low in micronutrients), glucose is not able to enter your cells and ends up staying in your blood as a result. This means your cells are starved of the fuel they need to operate, and signals are therefore sent to your brain to increase insulin. This results in cravings for sugar, because even though you may be eating enough, your cells are not able to access the food.

Food sensitivities: Food sensitivities are often the result of a situation known as 'leaky gut', where partially digested food particles can make their way into the bloodstream through a damaged, inflamed mucosal lining in the digestive tract. The body regards these food particles as foreign antigens and mounts an immune response by sending antibodies. Combined antibodies and antigens in your bloodstream, known as immune complexes, can lead to intense cravings. Gluten may be at the root of this type of sugar craving because it is often combined with sugar in the foods we eat, and so women think they are craving sugar when really they might be craving gluten.

Intestinal yeast or systemic candidiasis: Yeast thrives on sugar (a connection easy to make when you look at the Latin name for this group of organisms – saccharomycotina – or 'sugar fungi'). If your intestinal (and vaginal) bacteria are out of balance, they are less likely to keep yeasts like candida in check. An overgrowth of yeast - in the intestine or system-wide - can lead to increased cravings for sugar.

A lack of sweetness in your life (too much savoury!)

As I mentioned before, many things in life can affect our serotonin and beta-endorphin levels – exercise, balanced nutrition, rewarding work, a positive relationship, and even a sunny day. The joy we find in our lives speaks to our biochemistry. Therefore, when we are lacking positive energy and happiness, it's not surprising that we seek to fill that void with sugar. Life is about balance, when we tip the balance we see adverse results. So go on – inject some sweetness back in!

Chapter notes:

Many women engage in emotional eating;

Sugar acts like a drug;

Stress is a significant factor in emotional eating and sugar cravings.

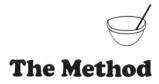

The Method

This method has come out of years of dieting, using my body and my clients' bodies to find an easy-to-follow dietary lifestyle that works long-term.

I have a history of yo-yo dieting; I understand what it is to have a big emotional attachment to food. I have starved myself, binged on packets of biscuits, sweets and chocolate to the point where I would lie awake at night crying because I felt bad at what I had done. I would vow to myself that tomorrow was a new day, a fresh start and then I would just repeat the same behaviour.

I have created a method that ends the guilt, you will no longer feel bad about treating yourself to nice foods and you will stop the obsession with food.

So how does it work?
Six Pack Chick works by balancing out blood sugar. When you eat lots of refined carbohydrates you feel full of energy for a short while, and then you slump back down again and need more sugar to perk yourself back up. I lived like this for years, getting fatter and more irritable every day.

An example of this is a snapshot of my old eating habits:

Breakfast (usually around 9.00am)
Granola with semi skimmed milk – honey coated cereal;
Freshly squeezed orange juice;
Latte with teaspoon of sugar;

I used to **LOVE** this breakfast and felt it used to give me loads of energy.

Mid morning
Piece of fruit – banana or apple;
I would be really hungry mid morning and crave something sweet.

Lunch (usually around 1.00pm)
Sandwich from the supermarket – cheddar cheese ploughman's used to be a favourite;
Bag of reduced fat crisps – found out they may have had less fat, but they were full of sugar;
Fruit yoghurt – they may have bits of fruit in them but they also have sugar, too.

Mid afternoon (usually around 3 or 4pm)
Coffee and small bar of chocolate;
I always used to have an energy slump; sometimes I just wanted to sleep and would often be really cranky.

Dinner (usually around 7.30pm)
Supermarket ready-meal, like chicken wrapped in Parma ham;
Mashed potatoes;
Roast vegetables;
I loved mashed potatoes and would always try to have vegetables with my dinner. I realised that my chicken ready-meal had lots of hidden sugar in the sauce.
Tried never to have dessert

Late evening
Couple of pieces of dark chocolate;
Unable to resist something sweet anymore, I would break off a couple of squares of chocolate hidden in the fridge.

Later evening
Fruit yoghurt or a biscuit;
Would watch TV and want to snack on something, usually driven by
food advertising on TV or just because I wanted something sweet to
munch on and treat myself after a hard day.

What I know now is that this is a classic example of my unstable blood
sugar. I would yo-yo up and down like this every day, feeding my sugar
craving several times a day.

Some symptoms of low blood sugar are as follows; see if you recognise
any of them in your day:
Shakiness; anxiety; nervousness; headache; palpitations; irritability;
feeling cold, and clammy hands.

There are other symptoms but these are the most common.
With my method, you will be filling up on foods that prevent low
blood sugar from happening. You will go through your day without
the dips and huge cravings for snacking on sugary junk. You will think
far less about food.

You will also learn the difference between true hunger and cravings.
Most of us do not recognise true hunger. Food is an emotional trigger,
so we tend to satisfy our cravings as and when we get them. This
emotional response will stop and you will make good food choices and
never feel guilty or 'chained' to food ever again.

OK, so what can I eat?
The Six Pack Chick *method is simple.*
You will eat proteins, pulses and fats six days a week. One day a
week, you will have 'treat' day. After your usual breakfast, you can eat
whatever you like. Yes, you read that right.

WHATEVER YOU LIKE

Try and resist the temptation to turn straight to the chapter Explain treat day; all will be explained as you work your way through the book!

Foods and drinks to choose:
Protein
Here is a list of all the proteins you can include:

Meat	beef, pork, lamb, veal, offal;
Poultry	chicken, turkey, duck, goose, guinea fowl, pheasant, all eggs;
Veg. protein	tofu, tempeh, quorn.

Carbohydrates

Pulses	lima beans, aduki beans, miso, black beans, mung beans, black-eyed peas, navy beans, fava beans, peas, garbanzos, split peas, kidney beans, pinto beans, lentils (green, red, yellow, puy, etc.), soy beans.
	Miso, tempeh and tofu are all derived from the soy bean, and are particularly good for vegetarians/ vegans.
Vegetables	most vegetables, apart from root vegetables i.e. potato, sweet potato, carrots, swede, turnip, parsnip;
Fruits	avocado, tomato.
Fats	Coconut, macadamia or extra virgin olive oil; Butter; Cream (limit to 1 dessert spoon in a coffee).

Drinks

Plenty of water   I cannot stress this enough. With removing
refined carbohydrates and grains from your diet,
constipation can be a temporary side effect. Six to
eight glasses of water a day as a standard, plus extra
if you are exercising.

Herbal teas;
Tea and coffee;
Red wine   (1 glass a day) The reds lower in sugars are best like
Zinfandel, Cabernet Sauvignon, Syrah, Pinot Noir.

Foods and drinks to avoid (six days a week)

Grains: amaranth, barley (pot or pearl), bulgur wheat, cornmeal,
couscous, cracked wheat, durum wheat, millet, oats, popcorn, rice (all
kinds), rye, spelt, wheat.
Every kind of bread - crackers, biscuits, cakes, pasta (penne, spaghetti,
etc.) and noodles - is made from grains.

Fruits: All fruits apart from avocado and tomato.

Sugars: The most common names for sugar are: barley malt, corn
syrup, dextrose, fruit juice concentrate, glucose, high-fructose corn
syrup, maltodextrin, maltose, molasses, raw sugar, sucrose, caster
sugar, icing sugar, granulated sugar, brown sugar, Demerara sugar,
fructose, honey.

Alcohol: All alcohol apart from red wine (1 small glass a day).
Drinks: Fruit juices, fizzy drinks, cordials, mixers, smoothies,
milkshakes.

Here is a 'watch list' for sugars that are hidden in many processed foods:

Agave nectar
Barbados Sugar
Barley malt
Beet sugar
Blackstrap molasses
Brown sugar
Buttered syrup
Cane crystals
Cane juice crystals
Cane sugar
Caramel
Carob syrup
Castor sugar
Confectioner's sugar
Corn syrup
Corn sweetener
Corn syrup solids
Crystalline fructose
Date sugar
Demerara Sugar
Dextrin
Dextran
Dextrose
Diastatic malt

Diatase
D-mannose
Evaporated cane juice
Ethyl maltol
Florida Crystals
Free Flowing
Fructose
Fruit juice
Fruit juice concentrate
Galactose
Glucose solids
Golden sugar
Golden syrup
Granulated sugar
Grape sugar
Grape juice
concentrate
HFCS
High-fructose corn
syrup
Honey
Icing sugar
Invert sugar
Lactose

Malt syrup
Maltodextrin
Maltose
Mannitol
Maple syrup
Molasses
Muscovado sugar
Organic raw sugar
Panocha
Powdered sugar
Raw sugar
Refiner's syrup
Rice Syrup
Sorbitol
Sorghum syrup
Sucrose
Sugar
Syrup
Table sugar
Treacle
Turbinado sugar
Yellow sugar

(Phew...what a list!)

OK, so you are probably thinking that I am part of some 'anti-sugar' brigade. From my experience with hundreds of clients, I believe that sugar is the cause of many of our problems in modern society. It acts like a drug for me. I cannot just have one biscuit, or a small piece of cake or a small square of chocolate, and I don't know many people who can. As a treat, it is fine but most of us don't know where that cut off point is; I certainly don't. It does not matter how full I am, I can **ALWAYS** have room for dessert in a restaurant.

Banning myself from it forever didn't work either and that is why I don't ban foods on this lifestyle programme. Once a week you are permitting yourself to have it, there is no pressure to never eat sugar again, no guilt associated to it when you do indulge on your treat day. That is why this method is sustainable; mixing a little bit of the bad with the good every week makes life more enjoyable and varied.

My top five foods

Through a lot of research and a whole lot of tasting, I have come up with the top ten foods to include in your new lifestyle:

Avocado: 'An Avocado a day keeps the wrinkles at bay' – these ought to be a 'super food'. Avocados are packed full of goodness and are my favourite food. I eat one every day. About 75% of an avocado's calories come from fat, most of which is monounsaturated fat. Avocados also have 60% more potassium than bananas. They are rich in B vitamins, as well as vitamin E and vitamin K.

Avocados have high fibre content among fruits – including 75% insoluble and 25% soluble fibre.

Coconut oil: I use coconut oil a lot. Apart from using it on my skin as a moisturiser, I use it as a hair mask, too. Once mistakenly believed to be unhealthy because of its high saturated fat content, research has shown that the fat in coconut oil is unique and different from most all other fats and possesses many health-giving properties. It is widely gaining recognition as nutritious oil recommended for cooking with. I use it to cook my eggs with in the morning and it is delicious.

Broccoli: Broccoli is high in Vitamin C, Vitamin A, folic acid, calcium and fibre. Not only is it a rich source, but half of its fibre is insoluble and half is soluble, helping to meet your needs for both types of fibre. Broccoli provides an added bonus in the form of protective substances that may shield you from disease. It is a cruciferous vegetable and it is widely known that an intake of cruciferous vegetables is linked to lower rates of cancer due to their phytochemical profile. Broccoli contains sulforaphane, which is a natural chemical that stimulates our bodies to produce enzymes and destroy carcinogens. This substance is particularly rich in broccoli sprouts and about 20 to 50 times richer in mature broccoli. It also contains a compound called indole-3-carbinol. This compound is said to reduce the risk of hormone dependent cancers such as prostate, breast and ovarian cancer.

Eggs: In praise of the egg –I eat two eggs every day. I love them. Best start to the day, especially on the Six Pack Chick lifestyle programme. In the past, eggs were thought to cause complications with cholesterol levels in the body. New studies show that eating two eggs per day can actually improve an individual's cholesterol levels. Eggs have approximately 5 grams of fat per whole egg, with only 1.5 grams being saturated fat.

Eggs are loaded with protein and a variety of minerals that are beneficial to the human body. One egg contains thirteen essential nutrients, including protein, choline, folate, iron and zinc. Eggs are also a great source of carotenoids (lutein and zeaxanthin), which have been shown to prevent macular degeneration in the eyes. In addition, eating eggs has also been shown to reduce the risk of developing cataracts.

I am a big fan of Burford Brown eggs; they are available in most supermarkets now and have beautiful dark brown shells and rich dark yolks. I will talk more about Burford Browns later.

Oily fish: – High in omega-3 fats (good ones!) oily fish are excellent Six Pack Chick food. Benefits of omega-3 oil consumption are:
- They reduce the levels of 'bad' LDL cholesterol in the blood.
- Omega-3 protects against heart and circulatory problems.
- Omega-3 is good for the development of a healthy baby, although pregnant women should limit themselves to no more than two portions of oily fish a week.
- Omega-3 may help patients with diabetes. People with diabetes often have high triglyceride and low HDL levels. Omega-3 fatty acids from fish oil can help lower triglycerides and apoproteins (markers of diabetes), and raise HDL, so eating foods or taking fish oil supplements may help people with diabetes.

Good sources of fish high in omega-3 oil are: sardines, mackerel, salmon, herring, and anchovies.

Physical benefits of the SPC method
These are from my observations with clients and from the trial group on Facebook:
- **Fat loss** – the results have been incredible. I lost 4.7 inches in three months. My waist is the smallest it has ever been. Out of 150 people in my trial group, this was the biggest and most widely reported benefit to the SPC method. One of my celebrity clients lost her 'baby weight' in two months, another client wanted to drop two dress sizes in a year. She did it in

three months. She is so happy with the result that she has continued with the method as she finds it so easy to manage and wants to carry on feeling as good as she does, eating the way she does.

- **More energy** – without the rollercoaster of high/low blood sugars everyone agrees that they have more energy. I sleep much less than I used to, and wake up raring to go every day.
- **No more bloating** – without refined sugar in the diet everyone agrees that the SPC method banishes the bloat!
- **No more headaches** – many people have headaches that are connected directly to low blood sugar. When blood sugar is balanced, there are no more headaches. I used to suffer particularly badly with headaches, sometimes migraine. I cannot remember the last time I had a headache.
- **Better concentration** – the SPC trial group all agreed that concentration was much better, adopting it very quickly into their new lifestyle. The brain feels much sharper, possibly due to the higher intake of omega-3.
- **PMT/PMS symptoms** greatly improved/disappeared – better balance of blood sugar and more stable mood.
- **Acne clear up** – one of my first problems to clear up was acne. I suffer from Polycystic Ovary Syndrome and cystic acne was a big problem for me. I haven't had acne since one month into the SPC lifestyle. I occasionally get a small spot but very rarely (one a month). Other clients who I have put on the method report the same benefit. Some fellow nutritionists and I all agree that acne should be re-named 'skin diabetes'. When the trigger is removed ie. sugar, the acne disappears. The higher intake of omega-3 helps the skin and acne scarring goes, too.
- **Shiny, healthy hair** – my hair started falling out when I came off the contraceptive pill. I had been on the pill for

fifteen years. It had completely masked my PCOS. My hair started falling out a lot, handfuls at a time. It has now thickened, and is really shiny and no longer falling out. As well as ingesting coconut oil, I also use it on my hair as a conditioning mask. Smells delicious, too!

There are many other benefits; you may find that inflammatory conditions get better, allergies like eczema and asthma improve, fungal infections like thrush clear up, your immune system is stronger and you keep viruses at bay.

Along with the physical benefits, there are psychological ones, too. For most women, yo-yo dieting is a way of life. You find a diet, try it, it works for a while and then you give up because it is too hard. Therefore, you go back to eating the way you did and just get fatter. The weight gain makes you feel depressed, like a failure and out of control. Sound familiar? This was a constant pattern for me and I just got more and more despondent.

The SPC method became all about getting rid of the guilt, removing that feeling of being obsessed and trapped by food.

Introducing Michelle Zelli

Michelle offers over fifteen years experience working in the field of human behaviour, science of the mind and coaching for success. With media appearances including Good Morning TV, BBC Radio and regular features in the national press, Michelle is renowned for getting results for her clients where everything else has failed. Her flexible approach offers a no-nonsense range of methods to cut through old patterns, fears and blocks to create the results you want.

Michelle is joining forces with me to launch my Six Pack Chick one-day events and not only has she been a fantastic coach to me, she is also now a great friend.

Psychological benefits of the SPC method

- No messing! No weighing! No counting! No hassle! Your mind loves to keep things simple!
- Routine! Your mind is programmed to work to habit. With SPC, you eat at regular intervals, with clear structure. Perfect!
- Positive re-enforcement. SPC gives fast results, feeding your mind with evidence of success as you quickly see yourself moving towards you goal!
- Empowerment. Feeling in control, where previously your eating habits controlled you. Now you have the power of your mind to create the shape you want!
- Success. With fast results showing in your mirror, your mind quickly demands more feel good factor, driving you forward towards your goal.
- Mind food! No processed, unhealthy food intake allows your mind and body to be at its best, firing on all cylinders. You enjoy energy and focus like never before!
- Breaking the rules! Your mind loves to rebel and by having a cheat day every week, eating everything you love and desire, you can relax knowing your day of decadence and reward is just around the corner!
- Permission is granted! Your old pattern of feeding on guilt and shame is a thing of the past, with cheat day you have absolute permission to indulge your culinary senses to the max and still feel good, stay in control and get results!
- Support. Every human needs to feel that they belong, as your

mind craves connection. With the SPC support network, real-time, you are encouraged, loved and nurtured throughout every stage of your journey.

- Simply feeling good! Your subconscious mind is designed to move towards whatever gives you the greatest pleasure, comfort and certainty. Great news! SPC works fast, allows a varied diet and a cheat day, fulfilling every feel-good factor. Looks, body shape, health and naughtiness are all catered for. You have it all.

Chapter notes:

- You will enjoy protein, pulses and vegetables;
- You can have a glass of red wine every day;
- You will get one day a week to enjoy all your favourite foods (and you get to read all about that in just a second);
- You will have energy, reduced mood swings and will change your relationship with food into a positive mindset.

Treat day – mixing the naughty with the nice

I came to the conclusion a long time ago that it was completely unrealistic to eat like a nutritionist saint for the rest of my life. I used to start off the day with all the best intentions in the world and eat really healthily, and then blow it all towards the end of the day when I was hungry, miserable and tired.

If you love eating a certain food, why on earth would you want to give it up for the rest of your life? The moment you tell yourself you are not allowed to eat something anymore, I can guarantee you will obsess about that food every second, minute, and hour of the day. It just **DOESN'T** work.

I started off designing the SPC method by trial-eating all the foods on the 'foods to include' list and then treating myself once a day to something. The problem with doing that is two-fold. One problem I found is that I would have one treat, this would lead to another and so on...the other problem was that by keeping treats in the house it was as if they were taunting me all day. I find it is better at the beginning of your new lifestyle with SPC to take all your 'cascade foods' out of the house and when you have your first couple of treat days – go out and enjoy them. I bet you can tell me right now what your cascade foods are? Cascade foods are those foods that you can't just have one of. Mine include any nuts, Pringles (what IS it with those things?), chocolate biscuits and piping hot toast.

I then tried eating all the right foods for 60% of the week and allowing 40% of the week to eat whatever I liked. This did not work either, as I slowly changed the percentages until I spent 40% of the week eating the right things and 60% eating the rest.

Therefore, I set about keeping it simple and easy to follow, so I thought about treat day.

I like calling it treat day because I don't like the word 'cheat'. 'Cheat' has negative connotations and SPC is all about feeling successful, positive and guilt-free.

Several leading experts agree with my principles. If you have heard of the author Tim Ferris, he is one of my heroes. He brought out a book called The Four Hour Work Week and later brought out a book called The Four Hour Body. His principles are very similar to mine. At first when I read it, I was cross that I hadn't released my book before him (in a nice way!), however, I highly respect him and his work and one day I want to meet him. Tim, if you are reading this book, let's make it happen! He is part of a leading movement that agrees that taking one day a week to eat what you like, works.

This is why I like SPC Treat Day:

Psychological Benefits

- We all need something to look forward to – SPC Treat Day gives you something to look forward to. The method is easy to follow for the rest of your life. Once a week you are permitting yourself to eat exactly what you like, after your protein breakfast if you want to eat an entire bakery then you can. Alternatively, if you have a party you can go and enjoy it without saying no to champagne and canapés or sticky toffee pudding.

I don't know about you but I would go to parties and start off by being really good, passing on the crisps and picking up the healthiest thing I could find...when what I really wanted were the crisps, knowing full well that if I ate one, I would eat the entire bowl. Now I do not worry about that; I go to a party on treat day and REALLY enjoy it, with no guilt whatsoever.

- Rewarding a good week – there is something very satisfying about following the SPC method and you will see this when you start. When you get to treat day and you are feeling great, you really enjoy it. You reward your good effort and renewed energy by eating something that you really love. You begin to appreciate those treats more and enjoy the texture and taste of it far more than if you ate it every day.

There are also physical benefits to be had from treat day...yes, your eyes are not deceiving you!

- You need the metabolism spike – one thing you will notice from eating more protein, pulses, vegetables and healthy fats is that after a while you will eat less. One problem with some of the more extreme dieting methods is that you eat so few calories that your metabolism slows down dramatically. The moment you give in and start eating normally again, you pile on the body fat and end up heavier than you were before. I certainly found this. I could not sustain a very low calorie intake; I was so tired and hungry that I would blow it and binge for days and get fatter and fatter (and more miserable). In this new lifestyle, you will end up eating slightly less because you are feeling less hungry. Treat day causes your metabolism to be fired up once a week and you actually lose more body fat as a result.

Another hero of mine is Tom Venuto. Tom is a bodybuilder and superb nutritionist. His book Burn the Fat, Feed the Muscle is a food and fitness bible for many of his followers. He talks a lot about calorie cycling, this method works, too, but more for men who like their calculations and spreadsheets. I became too obsessed with working it all out but his principles are excellent and, if you have a boyfriend/ husband who loves working out and wants a ripped body, then Tom Venuto's book is a must-read.

OK, so I hear you saying..."Just how bad can I be on Treat Day?" Here is an example of the perfect SPC Treat Day for me:

9.00am	Wake up (always excited at the prospect of Treat Day).
9.15am	Do twenty-minute Six Pack Chick Six exercises (www.youtube.com/sixpackchicktv).
10.00am	Prepare omelette with two eggs, organic bacon and garlic mushrooms.
11.00am	Let the treat day commence!
11.01am	Large latte with chocolate croissant and a lazy look at the newspapers.
12.00pm	Take the dog for a walk.
1.00pm	Pick up magazines from lovely Mr Patel on the way back from dog walk.
1.15pm	Put the fire on and plump up the cushions on the sofa.
1.30pm	Make a cheese toasted sandwich (inspired by Fernandez and Wells in Soho who make the BEST cheese toastie in the world).
1.45pm	Collapse on the sofa with dog stretched out in front of the fire, while munching cheese toastie and reading magazines.
2.45pm	Oooops forget to feed the dog, after seeing her staring at my empty plate for fifteen minutes.
3.00pm	Jump back on sofa with a packet of Percy Pigs and watch a chick-flick.
4.30pm	Cuddle the dog, and sob at movie ending.

6.00pm	Suggest to boyfriend that we go for dinner (hint at romantic promises) and get him to book something.
8.00pm	Get dolled up and enjoy a **HUGE** pizza with several glasses of red wine.
10.00pm	Waddle home and take the dog for her evening walk with boyfriend, while holding hands (**HIS** attempt at romance).

The rest I leave to your imagination...

You will have an idea in your mind already about your perfect treat day. Close your eyes for a minute and imagine it, and walk through it in your thoughts. Feels good doesn't it? You are going to feel like that every week for the rest of your life – brilliant!

At the beginning of my new journey I maxed out my treat days, and I really went for it. Partly for experimental reasons as I wanted to see what the next few days' results were. What I find now is that I do not feel the need to go quite so crazy. I am almost into a year of my new lifestyle and often I forget to have a treat day. I realise that I was totally addicted to sugar for many years. It caused so many of my health problems throughout my twenties. Sometimes the day after treat day (at the beginning), I would get a flare up of some of my old symptoms: migraine, itchy skin, aching joints, depression to name but a few. Now my treat days mainly consist of fresh fruit, pasta and rice. I no longer crave the biscuits and cakes but I still love chocolate and make sure I include that.

The more you get used to leaving sugar out of your diet, often, the worse you feel after treat day. Sugar triggers so many problems for me now, therefore, I try to avoid it. Try jotting down how you feel for up to two days after a treat day; it's interesting to look back on it.

I like to spoil myself on treat day, not only in the food sense but also in other ways. I have become so much more aware of my skin, how I spend my time, what I do on my 'day off'. I used to spend so long thinking about food and now I just get on and enjoy life.

Some suggestions of things to do on treat day:

Hot bath with scented candles and essential oils.

A walk somewhere new – call a friend and go and take a walk somewhere beautiful, peaceful and new. It does not cost anything and really does leave you feeling happy and refreshed, physically and mentally.

Watch an old film – pick a classic film that you have not seen but have always wanted to. Nothing violent or overly sad. You cannot beat a feel-good classic movie.

Create a vision board. This is great to help focus your mind on the things you want to get out of life. Flick through some magazines and cut out inspiring images, places to visit, your dream home or a recipe to try. Stick them on to a big piece of coloured card and display somewhere prominent. This is a great way to remind yourself of the things you are aiming for.

Safety in numbers – the Facebook Group

One of the bonuses of some of the successful diet clubs out there like Weightwatchers and Slimming World is that people feel part of something. They feel like they belong to a community. If you have tried one then you will know what I am talking about. In the group are a bunch of people with many of the same fears and goals as you have.

They work very well and although I do not agree with some of the principles, I do acknowledge that for many people, these clubs are effective. I like to surround myself with people who share common goals with me. The power of a group is incredible and you form new friendships and support each other on your journey.

Connection is one of the six human needs – the feelings of belonging, and being understood. Having like-minded people to share the ups and the downs with, makes everything more fun.

It is great to meet up once a week and for some people, the accountability keeps them going, the fear of turning up and not having lost any weight is too much to bear. This is, however, one of the big problems that I have with this method. I was horrified to discover that people weigh themselves once a week. That was enough to put me off ever going ever again. The humiliation and guilt I felt when I was not losing weight fast enough made me very depressed. I hate scales, tape measures, in fact, I hate anything that involves numbers...they become an obsession and do not tell the whole story.

When I started writing the SPC method, I wanted a group that could encompass all of the benefits of a club, with no judgemental weighing and measuring each week. Where group members could support each other, swap recipe ideas and give each other a big high-five each time their waistbands got looser or they managed to get their skinny jeans further than above the knee.

The eureka moment

I was sitting in my office chatting on Facebook when I suddenly had a eureka moment. You know that moment, when suddenly a thought comes into your head that is so strong it pings you between the eyes. I was going to put Six Pack Chick on Facebook and I would set up a secret trial group so that people could join it and not worry about all their hopes and fears being aired for the world to see.

It started off as a trial group. I invited six friends, who I knew wanted to change their relationship with food (they are now called the Six Pack Chick Six!). I gave them all the knowledge to start them off on the method and I supported them through their first couple of weeks with regular messages and encouragement. Once they started to see results, I set about making it a proper trial group. I had people in there from 20–67 years old, all with different health problems, all wanting to lose weight and change their relationship with food.

(Understanding that not everyone likes Facebook, I suggest using it in a way that makes you feel comfortable. If you are really concerned, then set up an account in a different name and don't share any of your details publicly.)

After a couple of weeks, the group was flourishing. Every day people were posting up results and the excitement was growing:

"Hey you guys :) 7kg lost in 6 SPC weeks :) had a run in with a portion of chips (my downfall) on treat day and feel myself waving goodbye to

things I thought I'd be obsessed with forever... SPC Freedom – never felt better. x"

"Morning all! Since this diet, I have felt fantastic. I have more energy; sleeping much better and I am losing weight. People are starting to notice, which I love: D, some days I have my protein breakfast but when it comes to lunch I am not hungry Is that right ?? Oh and it's my treat day today and to be honest there is nothing I could say I really fancy lol, but sure I will find something. xxx"

"OK; I have lost about 9lb; 2cm off waist (the BIG problem), 2.5cm off bum; 3cm off chest. I have spent a bit longer doing my two-weeks getting started – having gone to seed over the wedding weekend, but back on track since then."

"I'm very pleased with progress so far (in fact, I'm feeling chuffed with myself!). I like the fact that I can eat a lot of things like eggs, pulses and meat, and can make myself feel very full as a result. The feeling of being full lasts an incredibly long time."

"The lack of sugar in my diet stops cravings; when I go into cafes it feels strange to look around and think 'there's not one thing in here I can eat'. Mostly, at least so far, I don't want to eat the 'not allowed' stuff I would have been living on three weeks ago. I am a man who has kept London's station cafes and food counters in business for decades, so it is fabulous to be free of the compulsion to constantly eat stuff: blood sugar, it seems, saps will power, not personality failings!"

"I don't mean to go on about this (but I'm just so thrilled I can't help myself!). Total cm loss in week 7 (I think!?); 10cm off my waist, and 8cm off both my chest and my hips! And I will shut up about it now (for today at least)!"

These are just a snapshot of the hundreds of comments in the secret trial group. You will have your own when you jump in and get involved. Nothing gives me greater pleasure that to watch someone who came in with a history of obsessing about food, turn it around and become so positive about their body that they could burst with happiness. It makes me excited to get up every day knowing that I am able to help many more people than my one-to-one clients.

Facebook is the biggest social networking website of its kind; my aim is to outgrow it eventually and have our own SPC social network!

Connecting people from across the world

One of the things I love about Facebook is that you can connect with people from all over the world. It is like having 24/7 group therapy in our secret trial group. You might be awake in the middle of the night and struggling with something – you post up your question and someone answers immediately. You do not have to wait a week until your next meeting. You get an answer from someone who knows how you are feeling and gives suggestions on how to deal with it.

People have made great new friends in our group, firm bonds have been established and often new friends meet up and share treat day together or cook an 'SPC-friendly' meal and invite other group members around.

Because SPC is a lifestyle and not a quick fix diet, you know that people are in it for the long run and so it is not a constantly changing group. The Six Pack Chick Six are still in there and some of them post every day.

Common interests

I discovered in the early days of the group how Six Pack Chick is perfect for connecting new mothers. So many members join the group when they have just had a baby. Tired and uncomfortable with their post baby body, they come into the group to discover many other women in a similar position. The SPC method works brilliantly for new mothers and the results are very fast. One group formed a mini sub group called the SPC New Mums which meets up twice a week for a brisk walk and a chat to share recipes **AND** baby tips.

A couple of group members are athletes who need to strip body fat for long distance running and triathlons. I know they also meet regularly both on Facebook chat and for a run in the park. They support each other in their fat loss goal and in their sports.

Support and encouragement

I have already touched on this but it needs saying again! The greatest benefit of the group is the support.

If you are having a rubbish day, or you are not clear about what you are doing, you can go on, post it up there, and guarantee that several people will comment. One example of this is here:

(Name removed)
"Oh I am 4 days in and just realised that I have been eating oats, silly me, I forgot we weren't supposed to eat grains. Have I completely ruined my efforts??????????????????????"

"Nooooo don't worry, it is all a learning curve at the beginning. Remember, this is a lifestyle and not a quick fix. You have the rest of your life to get it right and you are doing so well. Keep up the good work!!! Xxxx"

"Stay strong (name removed), we have all been there. After a couple of

weeks, it will be second nature and you won't even have to think about it. Ask as many questions as you like and we will help you!! Xx"

This response is fantastic; people are so kind and supportive and just want all the newbies to feel as great as they did at the beginning. You will find that too; get involved from day one and the group will help you with everything you need.

Equally, if you see a big change for the positive, people will high-five you all day long. This example is from Joanna Beale who I talk about in another chapter. She is one of the original six and has made astounding progress:

"Well done! As I told you, the changes are visible! You look great!"

"You looked very slim bean when I saw you on Friday :-)"

"Thanks you guys :)"

"That's over a stone! Fabulous! Well done you! X"

"Well done Joanna!!"

"Fantastic! Well done u!"

Six Pack Chick is one big 'Girl Power' network. Men are welcome, too (if they are happy to chat with thousands of women!!).

I am known in the group as Mother Hen, it is what a lot of my clients have always called me and now the group do too. I can often be found signing off a post 'MH xxx'.

Sign on the dotted line
and let's get started

One of the most important things apart from the group support online, is full support from your family and friends. If you are anything like me, they are probably fed up of hearing that you are on 'another diet'. They will roll their eyes and yawn, and inside, they will be wondering how long **THIS** one is going to last.

The first thing you need to tell people is that this is not a diet. This is a lifestyle method. Yo-yo dieting does not work and frustrates everyone around you when you have to be really careful, counting calories or living on cabbage soup and it is very antisocial.

I am giving you all the tools to have an easy to follow, lifelong way of eating that you can adapt to fit in with others' eating habits. Before we continue, there is one quick tip I want you to really think about right now:

TIP: Beware of the saboteurs.

These are the female friends who, when they see you progressing and losing body fat, automatically try and sabotage your efforts. It might be along the lines of, *"Oh go on, have just one biscuit, I will hide the rest"*, or, *"Don't lose too much weight, you won't look well"*. Sound familiar? I am very used to this and could write a whole book about it. You may be unhappy with your body right now, reading this, and therefore, I want you to surround yourself with people who are going to support you. You need friends and family to encourage your efforts and help you through the first couple of weeks. One of the best ways of doing this is to write them a letter.

You can write your own letter or copy this one if you find it a helpful template.

Dear...

This is a letter to explain that I am embarking on a dietary lifestyle, as I want to improve the way I eat and my relationship with food. I have started to get... (You can list your individual ailments or weight gain etc.) and I would like to do something about them.

I would really appreciate your help and cooperation with this and please understand that this is not a fad diet; it is a change in lifestyle for me. I am happy to bring food with me that I can eat so that I do not require you to cater for my individual needs but, if you are interested in what I am doing, I would be happy for you to read the book on the subject.

I am excited about my new lifestyle and thank you for helping me.

Bridget

If you do not want to tell people face-to-face what you are doing, or you have been invited away to stay at someone's house for a few days, it really helps to prepare them in advance. You will find that most people will be supportive and will almost certainly want to know more!

Beware of the 'expert' opinion

One thing I want to mention is suddenly everyone around you will become the expert. Often they will dish out old scare stories or say something that they have no evidence to back up. Here are a few examples with the answers I give when it happens to me:

'Expert opinion': You eat eggs for breakfast every day? Aren't they really high in cholesterol?

My answer: Yes, I love eggs in the morning. I have eaten two a day for the last year and my cholesterol is better than it has ever been. Scientists have now proven that moderate consumption of eggs does not alter the bad cholesterol levels. You can point them to this article if they need convincing further
http://www.bhf.org.uk/heart-health/conditions/high-cholesterol.aspx

'Expert opinion': So basically, you are totally cutting out carbohydrates? You need carbohydrates for energy; you will feel awful (This particular one really irritates me!)

My answer: Firstly, I am not cutting out carbohydrates. There are plenty of complex carbohydrates in vegetables and pulses and I actually find on the SPC method that I have more energy, not less. I had a real problem with refined sugar in the past, it made me feel bloated, I put on weight and was more tired, not less. I feel great eating the way I do now; you should try it! That is usually enough to shut them up.

'Expert Opinion': It sounds very similar to the Atkins diet; didn't he die of a heart attack?

My answer: It isn't really like the Atkins diet; I eat lean meat, fish, pulses and vegetables with plenty of essential fats and less saturated fat. It is much better for me than the Atkins diet, although I believe many people manage really well on that. I am doing a dietary method that I can sustain long-term.

'Expert Opinion': No Dairy?? Will you get brittle bones? Are you getting enough calcium?

My answer: My diet is high in green vegetables, especially things like broccoli and celery. Both are extremely high in calcium **AND** I get the antioxidant benefit of the vegetables, too. Not a problem for me.

OK, let me sign on the dotted line.....

So, now you are saying: "OK, OK Bridget, enough already. I want to start **NOW**."

Let me prepare you for your change in life and tell you how to help yourself.

Go grab a pen as you are going to sign your name on this page.

"I want to change the relationship I have with food. I am fed up with yo-yo dieting and obsessing about what I eat. I am going to make a few simple changes that will improve my health, help me shift stubborn body fat and put a smile back on my face."

Date:
Signed..

The Bucket List

Have you watched the film 'The Bucket List'? If not, watch it. It is highly inspirational.

A bucket list is a list of things you want to do before you die. Morbid? Not really, it helps you focus on the things you really want to do or achieve.

Six random things on my bucket list are:
- Meet Oprah Winfrey – quite possibly one of the most amazing women I have ever listened to. I would love for her to become a Six Pack Chick.
- Learn sign language fluently and use it to instruct exercise – I understand that medicine is moving on, but I would love to be able to converse properly with someone who is hard-of-hearing or deaf.
- Be totally self-sufficient for at least a year – live off the land. Later in the book you will see that I absolutely **LOVE** chickens, particularly Burford Browns. I will be keeping chickens later in the year **AND** growing my own vegetables.
- Visit Petra in Jordan – mystical and breathtakingly beautiful.
- Listen to Josh Groban live – he has the most beautiful voice. It makes the hairs on the back of my neck stand up. Every time he has come to the UK I have missed him.
- Grow a six-foot sunflower – mine never grow beyond knee height (yes I know, I want to grow vegetables, not looking promising is it?).

It does not matter what you want on your bucket list. It is your list, not anyone else's, so you can put down anything you really want. Fill in the next page of your book. It does not matter how silly they are, as this is **YOUR** moment, so get creative and write down everything you want to do!!

My bucket list

Prepare yourself for Day One

If you haven't done it already – go and get your ball of string.

Now I would like you to measure yourself with string. No scales;
No tape measures, just plain old string.

Take as many measurements as you want to; I recommend on top of
bust, waist, hips, widest part of arms, and the widest part of thighs.
Label the pieces of string and put them in a pretty box. These will be
your guide from now on, so keep them safe!

Pick something tight

I like being able to see progress with my clothes. I had a pair of skinny
jeans that I bought in the vain hope I could squeeze into them. No
chance – I could not even get them up past my mid thigh! I remember
being so depressed and hating myself at that precise moment. Now I
can laugh about it, especially as I can do them up and wear a belt ;-)

Pick some item of clothing as a target. Try to get it on and say to
yourself, *"I am not able to get into these now, but I will do in the
months to come."*

Prepare the cupboards and the fridge

I think of this as a good clean out before starting your new life. Clear
out all the junk food in the house. If you have a family then put all the
foods that you may have trouble with in one place, so that they are
not scattered all over. Clean out the fridge and organise everything.
Psychologically it makes you feel clean and ready for a new start and,
if you want to, you can give foods to a neighbour or friend or even take

a box of food to a homeless shelter.

Do not hide foods or get your partner to hide them. If you are anything like me, you will have the ability of a scent-hound to seek out the foods you shouldn't have.

Take the time now to compile a shopping list.

I organise mine into the categories that I need to fill; type out this list and save a copy of it on your computer and then simply circle the things you need to buy each week:

Shopping list

Meat (organic if possible)
Recommended:

- Lean minced beef;
- Lean minced pork;
- Lean minced turkey;
- Chicken breasts.

Other

- Lean beef steak;
- Duck breast;
- Any joint of meat (for Sunday roast or to cook and slice up for snacking).

Fish

Recommended:

- Packs of prawns;
- Smoked mackerel fillets;
- Smoked salmon or trout (cheaper);
- Fresh oily fish i.e. sardines (great on a BBQ).

Other

- Any fresh fish that you like...sustainable source!

Eggs

Recommended:

- Burford –Browns – wonderful orangey yolks and great taste.

Other

- Go for as fresh as possible. Omega enriched eggs are good, too.

Vegetarian foods

Recommended:

- Tofu;
- Tempeh (great snack);
- Miso soup;
- Soya mince.

Other

- Cauldron marinated tofu pieces – good snack food, already cooked and so easy to eat.

Vegetables

Recommended:

- Avocado (I have put it in this section as it is near the other vegetables in the supermarket);
- Broccoli;
- Celery;
- Cucumber;
- Peppers;
- Aubergine;
- Courgette;
- Dark green leafy vegetables like kale, cabbage;

- Fresh/frozen edamame beans.

Other

- All vegetables apart from root vegetables.

Tinned foods

Recommended

- Tinned tuna;
- Tinned sardines;
- Tinned salmon;
- All pulses, but make sure they are in water, no sugar or salt;
- Tinned lentils.

Frozen foods

Recommended

- Frozen fish fillets;
- Frozen –broccoli – flash frozen, so often more vitamins and minerals than fresh;
- Frozen peas;
- Frozen edamame beans.

Sundries

Recommended:

- Coconut oil;
- Macadamia nut oil;
- Chilli sauce (with no sugar);
- Smoked paprika;
- Sea salt;
- Fresh herb plants;
- Meat and fish rubs, or make your own with dried herbs and spices;
- Chickpea flour – use for dusting things to make them crispy!

- A nice bottle of Cabernet Sauvignon – some organic wines are really nice, and they are not expensive and don't contain sulfites. Bonus.
- Organic cream – some people don't like black coffee, so add a teaspoon of cream to it.
- Lemon – to slice and put in water or tea.

Drinks

Recommended:

- Herbal teas;
- Green or White tea;
- Diet coke – no more than one a day;
- Good quality coffee;
- Rooibos;
- Tap water is fine; no need for mineral water. (I am not keen on plastic bottles because of the impact on the environment as well as the implications of plastics on health. I recommend using a water filter jug and, if you are having dinner parties, then use a glass bottle instead.)
- Sense of humour (only kidding; imagine if you could buy **THAT** in a supermarket?).

What to expect in the first two weeks

I am going to keep this simple; here are some things that you might notice and solutions to deal with them.

You may experience weakness, low blood sugar, tiredness.

The solution is to make sure you eat enough. Most clients when they report this problem have not eaten enough. I will remind you that you are not calorie counting. You eat from the selected foods and must never get hungry. If you are hungry then you have not eaten enough.

Like me, you may crave sugar like crazy in the first week. I was dreaming about it. Sugar for me is like a drug, I went through horrible withdrawal and it was not helped by not eating enough. Have the breakfast, a mid morning snack, lunch, mid afternoon snack and dinner. It really does help, I promise!

Useful tip: If you get a bad craving for sugar, then dab some vanilla essence or vanilla perfume oil on the back of your wrist. It worked wonders for me; it fooled my brain into thinking I had eaten something sweet.

I also made the mistake of doing intense exercise in my first week. It is so typical of the old me – totally change the way I eat **AND** workout hard at the same time and expect my body to deal with it. Give yourself a break; just go for a brisk walk each day for at least 20 minutes. You will get fresh air and some exercise without exhausting yourself.

In the first seven days, I want you to start some simple visualisation. It really helps to target the body you want. It creates a positive frame of mind and I have just the person to help you.

Michelle Zelli's Visualisation

Do you see yourself as slim, healthy and happy? Are you ready to create the new you?

Every behaviour, habit or feeling you have often starts in the mind. Quite unwittingly, we have programmed our mind to focus on what we don't like about ourselves and see ourselves as unattractive, out of control or simply just unhappy about ourselves. By changing your focus, and using your mind to create different pictures, you have the power to fuel your motivation, increase your determination and transform the way you feel about yourself.

This simple exercise is an effective way to make instant shifts. Are you prepared to invest just 5 minutes twice a day to see incredible results?

* * * *

Sit comfortably, and make sure your phone is off and you will not be disturbed.

Close your eyes and take three deep breaths in through your nose, and then slowly exhale through your mouth. This practice will release your tension, negativity and stress with each out-breath.

Picture yourself looking fabulous; notice the shape of your ideal body. Take in every detail. What are you wearing? Notice the colours.

Now focus on the way the fabric feels against your skin. Allow yourself to enjoy the feeling.

Take a good look at yourself from head to toe...what is the expression on your face; are you smiling or laughing? Take it all in!!

Where are you? Notice your surroundings, and take in every detail.

Turn on your Technicolour, making your picture now colourful, vivid and bright – and in perfect focus.

Now look around you; who is there? See the expression on their faces as they look at you; perhaps they are speaking to you...hear what they are saying. Pay attention to every word. Are they congratulating you?

Are they telling you how fabulous you look?

Let yourself feel how it feels to look so good, to have others around you noticing your success.

Revel in the feel good factor, and allow that great feeling to permeate every part of your body.

＊＊＊＊

Remember, you are re-programming your mind, building your muscle of success. Just like working out in the gym; if you do it once, it might feel OK, but you won't see a difference.

Your mind is like any muscle in your body; keep working it out until it is toned and lean.

Repeat this exercise twice a day; when you have the method off-pat, feel free to use it in the shower, when you are brushing your teeth or putting your make-up on – make it part of your routine. It is simple, it is fast, it feels great and above all it fuels your success from the subconscious mind... the most powerful ally you could wish for!!!

The Hen House -
Heroines (and one hero)
– how this book was possible

There are many people who have helped me to become the person that I am today, but there are a few people who really inspired me to go on and help others. One day you may meet them but until then, let their stories inspire you as you start your own Six Pack Chick journey.
The first person I would like to introduce you to is Joanna Beale.
Jo came to me as a client a year ago in a terrible way. She had a history of yo-yo dieting and was at rock bottom. Jo has completely turned things around and is part of the original Six Pack Chick Six. She works with me now and, not only does she make me laugh until I cry, she is the reason why I love to help people turn their self-image around.

Jo's story

People often say that the struggle with their weight began in their adolescence, but I found that the actual struggle did not really begin until much later. Early on in secondary school I began to identify myself as the 'fat one' amongst my friends – a size 14 at the age of fourteen – and the journey towards obesity really just seemed to be a self-fulfilling prophecy that I rather unconsciously resigned myself to at this early age. It was hard, yes, but a struggle, no. I just settled into it, and rather lazily accepted that this was me, destined for a life of fatness; maybe if the time was right in later life, I might magically wake up to find myself thin. I ate a lot and exercised little, in fact, most days I actively avoided most kinds of activity. There was a girl in my class at school, who was constantly on a diet, and she would give me her lunch before morning registration, and I would eat all of it, despite not being hungry and only just having had my breakfast. If I had a packed lunch, I would also have a meal in the canteen with my friends, often eating the packed lunch in secret. I did not realise it at the time, but I packed as much food into my day as I possibly could – mainly because it was always preying on my mind. Every spare moment was an opportunity to eat, and that continued on and on for many years. Food was always there, no matter where I was, or what went wrong.

There were cruel comments as I got bigger and bigger over the years, some laced with genuine concern, others just there to hurt. One boy at my school nicknamed me 'Jabba the Hutt', which fortunately I did not understand at the time – it was a few years later when it made sense that it stung. On one occasion, I was asked why I did not want to be pretty; I think I may have answered along the lines of there being no real point. At my largest, people would stop me in the street and tell me that I was, "Really fat", which did not lend itself to building up my self-esteem in the least. Every comment, whether I answered it, shrugged it off, laughed or ran away – hurt! They were like pins stuck in me that I couldn't remove, and as the years went by, and I grew larger, more hurtful pins were driven deeper into both my body and my mind.

Having been brought up with a 'low fat diet' ethos, I believed that carbohydrates were a safe food group – even massively high carbohydrate foods could be completely fat free! It's not that I did not know how I was 'supposed' to eat; it was just that I found it so hard to focus on a balanced diet. I knew everything there was to know about portion sizes, food triangles, calories and vegetables. I could have advised the universe and still not have had any control over what I actually put into my mouth. I would make occasions to binge eat, mainly to justify the intake of large amounts of food. I would never eat too much in front of someone I had only just met – in fact, quite the opposite. Nevertheless, when I knew someone well, I would always do my hardest to get them to join me in my binging. Through more than 15 years, I never met anyone who could keep on eating after I was finished. The worst part for me was that I never really ever felt full until the point where I could fit no more inside me. Therefore, I would keep eating until I reached that point as often as I could. I don't know why, but it was compulsive – the point at which I would lose control was way before I touched any of the food. The hunger was never in my stomach, it would always rage within my own head.

I spoke to five doctors and three psychological counsellors over the years about the fear that I had regarding food – and every single one advised that I try a low fat diet. Two prescribed Orlistat, which didn't work for me on either occasion, as I simply found it further facilitated my desire and ability to binge eat unhealthy foods. I tried to explain that I knew the rules and I just couldn't seem to apply them – that this problem wasn't in my belly, that I was simultaneously both terrified and obsessed with food, but it always fell on deaf ears. Just another fattie with no self-control.

I steadily gained weight from my early teens through my twenties. A couple of times I managed to diet or exercise a stone or two away, but by my mid-twenties, I was over 20 stone and at my absolute biggest. I could not walk without waddling; I was always out of breath and, to top it all off, I had a very painful boil problem everywhere that my skin rubbed against itself. I had to wash all the time because I just got so sweaty and started to smell. I could not even paint my own toenails. I hated every single moment of my existence, but still, I kept eating, maybe even more so, because I was too scared to leave the house most of the time. It wasn't just the comments in the street and it wasn't just the effort of physically getting anywhere – it was the feeling that I wasn't worthy of existing in public, the sense that I was no longer even a person because I had reached a state of such extreme disgusting-ness. I found it increasingly difficult to raise my eyes to look in front of me because I was so deeply ashamed of how I must appear to the world. This inevitably led to stumbling, which in turn made my journeys outdoors even more embarrassing and, subsequently, even less frequent. I found that I associated my sense of self more with some of the names that I had been called than I did with anything that even resembled self-esteem. I was trapped in a self-fulfilling spiral because I believed all of those negative things more than I believed in myself.

Through that time, I became more depressed by the day. Personal circumstances, including a divorce and subsequent move, took me into a new environment and among new people. It wasn't until this point that I even realised what I had become. Seeing myself in another place only served to illustrate just how unhappy I was. My clothes were like sacks, my skin blotchy and sallow, but more than anything, after all that time I was finally confronted by the way that I felt about myself. One word summed it up: worthless. It was like having my heart broken a thousand times. I came face to face with every ounce of negativity in my soul and there was simply nothing else there. No denial, no nothing. A bleak emptiness that seemed to stretch out forever in front of me. And, so, I ate. That same week, my Dad remarried and many photographs were taken at his wedding. Whilst I would usually shy away from the camera, I was unable to on this occasion, and I had permitted the world and his wife to try to make me look in some way acceptable – something that I had pretty much written off as impossible. At the wedding, I overheard two members of my new stepfamily making fun of me in a language they thought I did not understand. In the same moment, a photograph was taken of me, and it is that picture that haunted every thought for many months afterwards. To see the photographs developed, and committed to an album to serve as memories for all time; to remember that moment when I heard them laugh; to feel the rising sickness of self-hatred that I had kept inside me all those years: that was the day that I had to change something.

Ironically, that was actually the day that the struggle began. Because my denial had perpetuated my weight gain for years on end, I had never really fought my weight before. However, that day, battle commenced. I embarked upon a restrictive meal-replacement diet as the quickest available fix – desperate to eliminate the fundamental problem in my equation: food. I have never experienced hunger like it. Desperate, aching hunger that stretched out over every single day and, with every day that my body got smaller, my obsession with food grew. I lost over ten stone that year, and finally experienced what it was like to be thin. Nobody recognised me and I felt as if I had truly achieved something. The problem was, it was not the glamorous life that I had always imagined. It not only hurt just to stand up and sit down, but I was dizzy every time I did. I had to wear two layers of foundation to disguise the fact that my skin had no colour, and I had to sleep fourteen hours a night just to have the energy to go to work. My hairline receded quite significantly, and all my joints ached constantly. I had reached the point where I was counting my calories so strictly, and recording them in such a detailed way that I had books and books full of data on what I had eaten, how much exercise I had done (ten hours minimum, or I would have to punish myself), my measurements, and my weights (both morning and evening).

Nevertheless, I could have put up with everything if I wasn't so totally consumed by the unending desire to eat. Every single thought was not just of food, but of self-denial – of a feeling that to eat was to fail, or was self-sabotage. Every stomach rumble was a test, which I passed for a couple of years. However, I felt myself getting weaker, and I knew that my control would slip, that I would fail, that it could not last this way forever. The nagging thought at the back of my mind was that of the fat girl hiding inside me. She might have been invisible now but she was always there, begging me to fill my stomach with all the food that she filled my mind with. I would dream every night of ice cream or crisps, bingeing in my sleep, until the moment I woke up feeling so guilty that I would deny myself breakfast.

Then, one day, it happened. I was baking cakes that I used to sell, enduring a torture that I subjected myself to every week just to prove how much I had changed. I ate one of them. And another. And another. And then, I licked the spoon, and the bowl. And ate another cake. Every bite frenzied and furious, as if forced by the hand of another. Tears streaming down my face I tried to make myself sick for half an hour, jamming anything I could find down my throat, but to no avail. A handful of laxatives and I tried to forget it had happened, but I could feel the weight in my stomach all day. I felt dirty, disgusting. I had failed; it had all been worth nothing. There I was, a fraud, in my own kitchen. My entire existence felt built upon lies. All of those people who had been impressed and inspired by my amazing weight loss – I had let every single one of them down – lied to each one. That was the point that I became fat again – in the space of five minutes.

It was as if a door had been opened that could not be shut – the struggle ensued but the difference now was that I was losing. The only way I could make myself sick when I binged was to drink a massive amount of alcohol very quickly, which I tried, but had to stop when I ended up in hospital. Of course, I didn't admit what had happened, but the paramedics were more than confused at the sheer volume of food in my stomach. Thereafter, I tried making myself sick by eating only food that I thought had gone off, but that didn't work. Then, I kind of gave up and just started eating in secret, sometimes fishing my food from the bin so as not to leave any evidence. There were days I prayed for an eating disorder, or even a serious disease that might stop me eating, any kind of intervention which might turn it around. Moreover, as my weight crept up again, I stopped associating myself with the thin girl and gave back my life to the overweight fourteen-year old who ate without thought.

When I became pregnant at the weight of 90kg, I was terrified of harming my baby by putting on weight in pregnancy, and consciously ate well throughout. After I gave birth, I had gained only 1kg. For me, that came as a shock – mainly because it was so easy to eat well when I was doing it to look after someone else. It filled me with utter sadness that I had never been able to do that for myself. For a few weeks, I was happy with myself and my body, so proud of it now, having seen what I had achieved. However, it soon gave way to a terror that I was now the only new mother carrying so much weight; that my child would suddenly fall victim to childhood obesity and it would all be my fault for not losing three stone immediately after his birth.

In addition, there was more struggling, more yo-yo-ing for nearly a year. When I heard about Six Pack Chick from a friend, I was first sceptical, and second, I was afraid. I was so scared that I might try this plan and fail, as I had failed all the previous times; that this might just be another yo-yo waste of time and even more of a struggle than I was currently enduring. But, the thing I feared the most was that this might be my very last chance – that if this didn't work, that the rest of my life would carry on with the turmoil of a never-ending obsession with food. That fear nearly kept me from reaching the point that I am at today.

After only a fortnight, my relationship with food had changed completely. I no longer thought about it endlessly, no longer fantasized about the next thing I would eat. No more 'head hunger', just the heeding of true hunger when it called. A new satisfaction upon eating and a sense of fullness without the bloated agony of a stomach stretched beyond capacity. The pain just went away, as if it was never even there, replaced with a clarity of thought and being that I never thought possible. Losing weight stopped being a priority as I stopped thinking about food and started enjoying my life. Happiness became a reality.

I never thought I could be free of the demons that had gripped me for my entire adult life, and I never dreamed that the solution could possibly be so simple – or so easy.

****

The second person I would like to introduce you to is Natasha Woolman. Natasha is a mother of two beautiful girls and is **ALWAYS** smiling. I had no idea she was so unhappy about her weight until she came to me for help. Natasha was at a stage in her life where she really wanted to transform her body, and transform it she has. She looks incredible.

Natasha Woolman's story

My battle with my weight started when I was a teenager. I grew up in the Caribbean among a privileged circle of beach babes. I was slim, but had a slight pouch and what I now refer to as Beyoncé thighs and a J-Lo bum, neither of which were en-vogue at the time. I grew self-conscious and developed unhealthy issues with my weight. I always covered up on the beach and constantly felt unattractive, comparing myself to my much slimmer and more popular friends. I tried all sorts of diets and slimming aids, including one actually called 'Aids' - but that product soon disappeared from the shelves in the 80s! I even starved myself whenever I could get away with it, and all with limited success.

I moved back to England at sixteen to finish my education and lived with my father's cousin and his wife and kids. I was not entirely happy there (in hindsight that was because I missed my family) and I started to eat, a lot! Copious amounts of crisps, chocolates, chips, burgers – all the foods I shouldn't have been eating. I grew from there, quite literally. I was a size 12 when I arrived in England and progressively grew to over a size 20/22 at my peak earlier this year. I managed to lose a stone or two in the mid 90s when backpacking through India after my father died when I was 23, but then who wouldn't! It all came back when we hit the western world again!

My weight stabilised when I was happy and then I really hit rock bottom when my mother died when I was 29. She was diagnosed with stage 2 colon cancer and, following successful surgeries, the cancer was removed and she was due home from hospital for Christmas. She died before she could come home and before I could get to her. I took this really hard and ate my way through my grief. I couldn't see this at the time and honestly, I think I am realising a lot just writing this. But I digress. I ate more through my pregnancies as I was sad to be having children without my mother and grew some more until I actually became resigned to the fact I was going to be fat.

I must add that I quit a 30–40 a day smoking habit when I found out I was pregnant and this made me comfort eat even more!

Faced with two beautiful daughters and a loving husband, it dawned on me that I had to do something and fast. I was slowly killing myself, increasing my chances of developing cancer like my mother, and heart disease and diabetes like my father, while potentially leaving my girls with no mother. The thought of this made me eat more!

I tried Weight Watchers and managed to lose a few pounds but as usual lost interest in weighing and measuring and tracking. Then I saw what SPC had done for Ingrid Amis while trialling it and I wanted to try it. I did and I love it.

It has totally changed my relationship with food. I no longer over eat and I have learned to listen to my body and understand my cravings and reasons for them, thereby overcoming them (most of the time!). I feel so healthy and energetic and positive – even my GP is impressed! The pièce de resistance? Dropping four dress sizes so far, and still shrinking in a happy, healthy manner. This is one happy Chick!!!

★ ★ ★ ★

The next person is my own personal hero, Jake. Jake's Mum came to me one day asking if I helped teenagers to get a better self-image and shift excess body fat. I love helping teenagers; I remember what the teenage angst feels like when you are carrying too much weight, get bullied and suffer with depression. Jake came to me with a lot to lose and a distorted relationship with food. The progress he made over the following weeks and months transformed him from an unhappy kid to a confident and strong teenager. I believe Jake will go on to help hundreds, if not thousands, of other teenagers and I really wanted him to share his story in this book and here it is:

Jake's story

The first time I was unhappy was when my parents got divorced. I was around twelve years old, and that was the moment it all went pretty much downhill. I started overeating, but did not notice it for another one or two years.

It kept getting worse and worse. The first time I actually noticed anything was when I started hearing snide comments from other people about me, but I did not care about what they said. It probably made a lot of things even worse for me, because I got even unhappier. Since that point I have done a lot of different diets. I started with a normal diet, such as eating less of the bad stuff (eg. chocolate, gummibears) and more of the 'good stuff'.

It worked for the first three or four days, but then it got too difficult and I started bingeing on sugar again.

Shortly after that, I started going on the scales every morning and noting it down. This method did help longer than expected and I kept losing weight but, as before, it went wrong again.

After a year or so, I was heavier than ever before and, having talked with my parents, decided that I should go to 'Wellspring'. Wellspring was basically a fat-camp. It helped for the time being, but as soon I stopped I gained all of the weight and **MORE**. Also when you are at a fat-camp such as Wellspring, they keep you away from your family. All you get is two phone calls and that is it.

Then, in December 2010 and January 2011, I reached the point at which I knew I had to do something. That Christmas I was in America and I ate a lot of junk food. At the end of the trip, I went on a scale and discovered I was over 20 stone.

One day my mum told me that Bridget Hunt was promoting her dietary lifestyle and she would like me to participate. At first, I was a little sceptical, and I still was after Bridget introduced me to SPC. In the first week, the only thing I was looking forward to was treat day. It was all I could think about – the longer you do SPC the easier it is to resist anything – from chocolate to ice cream and cookies.

Now even though I haven't reached my goal of a six-pack...I weigh fifteen stone. I have lost over five stone (30kg) in just seven months. After the weight-loss, the funniest part is to compare old pictures with new ones and I get a lot of inspiring comments, which help me to continue.

I hope that I can inspire thousands of people, especially kids and teenagers who are unhappy with the way they look.

Jakob Drees

* * * *

My last client is very representative of some of my celebrity clients. I have worked with lots of celebrities; I do not advertise my dietary services and they know they get 100% trust with me. I am not seen out jogging in a London park with them. I offer a very discreet service and the outside world just sees a healthy, confident and in-control person. Most of the women I see in the public eye have struggled with the pressure of staying slim, parties where lots of food is begging to be eaten, and media pressure, scrutinising every lump and bump on show.

I am not publicising the name of this person who has written her story, but the story itself is very common.

Client A

I remember the first time I realised that I had to watch what I ate. I was at stage school and one of the older girls at lunch was telling another girl that she had a casting the next week and she was going to eat as little as possible so that she looked 'a million dollars' for the casting.

I was twelve years old and it made me really think about how I could improve myself.

I wasn't really fat, I just had a little puppy fat, but I was already conscious of it. My Mum always gave me a treat when I got home, and my favourite was individual trifles. I remember them so clearly; they had bits of sponge, jelly, custard and whipping cream on top. They were my treat for getting through the day, a day filled with dance, drama, singing and **PRESSURE**.

It was not OK to be good enough; we had to be excellent and were constantly reminded that we would only succeed if we were the best. I guess it must be the same at academic schools; extreme control of your body starts when you feel the pressure, whether it is getting top grades or being the slimmest dancer.

So I started off by telling my Mum that I no longer wanted those trifles after school; she wouldn't let me out of the house without breakfast and so before long I was choosing a type of cereal, which I became obsessed with, eating each piece one by one, slowly, chewing every grain, hoping it would make me full.

I would skip lunch at school, often feeling really dizzy by mid afternoon and would resort to a coke to keep myself going or an apple, which I would cut up into little pieces.

By the time I was sixteen, I knew the calorie content of every food, and the panic that would wash over me if I was forced to eat something I hadn't planned for. In those instances, I would go to the toilet and make myself sick. It became so easy and felt so normal. I felt such euphoria when I was sick, like I had won. I was 100% in control of myself and no one could take that away from me.

No one ever suspected what I was doing, I was very slim but I was doing a lot of dancing and so my figure was put down to 'a dancer's body' and a 'fast metabolism'. I hid behind that for years.

I was recommended to Bridget through a friend of mine; a model. She had battled for years with negative self-image. Bridget rather reprogrammed her thought patterns with no airy-fairy technique other than trust and understanding. She understood what she had to eat to stay slim, strong and healthy and I needed to do the same. I had got to the stage where my periods had stopped and my GP was asking questions about my eating and I just ran away from her questioning and never went back.

I immediately felt at ease in my first meeting. It was meant to be 60 minutes but I ended up talking, sobbing and laughing for three hours. Bridget did not stop me rambling on, and instead, she just listened. As I was talking I felt ridiculous, I sounded so extreme in what I had been doing to myself. Just saying it out loud for the first time shocked me and that was the day I turned round my life.

I saw Bridget only a handful of times; I stuck to her method and I put on some muscle, my skin cleared up, my hair started to look glossy and I no longer went through my day-to-day life feeling like I was in thick fog.

I consider myself to be one of Bridget's secret chicks. I am in the Facebook group under a different name and I love the support and understanding I get from the others. I don't post much but I log on every day and gain strength from every one's posts on there. I am trying to get pregnant and I know that when that happens I will be in control of my diet in a positive way; I will be able to eat healthily and support myself through pregnancy and know that I will shift any excess weight I may gain, in a safe way.

I will always remember my first session with Bridget and it is marked in my diary; 26th November 2010 – the new beginning.

Chapter notes:

- There is always someone out there with similar feelings to you.
- No matter how bad a person's eating history, it can **ALWAYS** be changed.

The Chicken Coop

Here in the chicken coop you will find tips and tricks, recipes, a dinner party menu, recommendations for how to follow SPC when you are out and about.

Tips and tricks
Walking

OK so I am a big believer in walking, I like to walk everywhere but I like to walk with a purpose – a great reason to get a dog. You may not have the lifestyle to suit a dog but you can always offer to walk a friend's dog, or failing that, ring up a friend and instead of nattering for an hour munching through a bag of crisps (something I used to do a lot), keep the call short and offer to meet him/her for a walk. If you chat away, you can walk for a good hour without even realising that you are exercising. I find my best recipes, ideas, and moments of clarity come when I am walking.

Having a pet is a big responsibility; all of you who have them will know what I am talking about. If you have ever thought about getting a dog, I can highly recommend it. Not only do you exercise every day but, I find just sitting and stroking my dog is a great stress reliever. I am a big fan of Lurchers and I have rescued two from an amazing charity called Lurcher SOS. They do not need a **HUGE** amount of exercise, and are very loving and just enjoy sleeping all day.

Girly evening

A girly evening does not need to be an all out binge on sugar and fatty snacks. I used to have those quite frequently and would always feel terrible the next day. When other people surround you, and there is a pile of junk food on the table, it is very hard to resist; so why not do a girly evening with a difference?

Have a healthy one:

1. **DVD that is either funny or inspirational. Do not watch something depressing or scary.**

2. **Pile of magazines – get each friend to bring a different one and swap when you have read yours.**

3. **Face mask – always makes me laugh. I remember doing this as a teenager and giggling uncontrollably when we put them on. The mud ones used to set and that cracking feeling you get when you smile is great. You can get them in sachets for 99p. Or, try these recipes for a fab home-made luxury face mask:**

Dry skin – mash half a very ripe avocado (you can eat the other half) with a tablespoon of honey. Mix well and apply to cleansed face with the back of a teaspoon. Leave for 20–30 minutes and rinse off.

Sensitive or sun burnt skin – mix two tablespoons of oatmeal with 1–2 tablespoons of live natural yoghurt and a teaspoon of honey. After mixing, apply to the skin with the back of a teaspoon. Leave for 20–30 minutes and rinse off.

Acne prone skin – destalk 5 ripe strawberries and add to food processor with a tablespoon of live natural yoghurt and an inch of peeled cucumber. Blitz well until smooth. Apply to the skin with the back of a teaspoon. Leave for 20–30 minutes and rinse off.

Watch You Tube and get some make-up tips. Great make-up is something that I still have not completely mastered but I am much better at it, thanks to Hanadi Hassanyeh. She taught me two simple looks – one for day and one evening look. You can search on You Tube for thousands of make-up lessons and it is a great fun thing to do on a girly evening.

Have a 'Stitch and Bitch' evening

A very good friend of mine holds these; four people get together once a week at a different house each week on rotation. They cook together and then do something creative. Some knit, some make hand-made greetings cards, and some make cushions. It doesn't matter what you make or if it is any good. It's about getting together with friends and doing something creative. Why not get three friends involved in Six Pack Chick and each cook an SPC friendly meal? You can invent and swap recipes that way.

Mother Hen Recommends
– how to eat out

Here are some recommendations for you, they are not essential but are a few things that I either love or really help on your Six Pack Chick journey.

Eating on the high street

One question that comes up time and time again with clients is: *"How am I going to eat lunch, as I normally go to a supermarket and just grab a sandwich?"*

Actually, it isn't that hard. I promise.

All you have to do is change your way of thinking; if you have the time and energy to prepare lunch and take it with you then great. I know a lot of people who simply can't get their head around this. Often I am too busy, or I forget and so need to stop somewhere and eat.

One of the problems that Six Pack Chicks face is that many of the coffee shops do not have **ANYTHING** that does not contain bread, pasta or rice. This is probably because these ingredients are cheap and are filling. My goal is to have SPC friendly meals in **EVERY** high street chain, and my own range of meals in the supermarkets.

Here are some suggestions that I use when I am out and about and in a hurry:

Prêt a Manger

I am so looking forward to the day that Prêt a Manger do a SPC salad box, as they **ARE** one of the better high street chains to get lunch. My three favourite options that they do currently are:

No Bread Crayfish and Avocado

Layers of wild crayfish and avocado, on a bed of salad leaves, served with a separate little pot of French dressing, so you can enjoy your lunch dressed or undressed! A pick-me-up of protein, vitamins B12 and C and selenium (great for glowing skin). You will feel fuller for longer (no grazing) and have more energy all from this delicious low-carbohydrate lunch.

Spanish Chorizo and Butterbean soup.

Smoky Spanish chorizo provides this soup with a real flavour of the Costa del Sol! We use huge butterbeans and combine onion, celery, rosemary, thyme and sage, and add a touch of chilli for a meal, which is fit for King Carlos himself.

Lentil and Smoked Bacon Soup.

This traditional soup is slow-cooked and hand stirred, which is arduous due to the sheer size of the saucepan, but worth it due to its sheer scrumptiousness. Soft lentils, rich smoked bacon flavour, and herbed goodness make a chunky soup that truly warms the cockles.

Nandos

Well what can I say about Nandos?? OK, so I wouldn't recommend that you eat here every day but there are days when only a trip to Nandos will do.

A lot of the things they do are SPC friendly.

Here is my suggestion (hopefully, you like chicken...).
Order a ¼ or ½ chicken with hot marinade (or extra hot if you dare).

Order a portion of ratatouille to go with it and a side salad. Filling and oh so delicious.

Tossed

One day I hope there will be a Tossed cafe in **EVERY** high street. Whenever I am in London, I go in there and buy one of their delicious super-fresh salads. They create a salad for you and you can make an SPC power lunch that keeps you full all afternoon.

Here is what they stand for:

"Following months of travelling the world in search of the perfect salad, not to mention weeks of tasting lettuce, leaves and healthy fillings, we opened our first store in Paddington, West London in April 2005. Our mission: to create a new, healthy and exciting food experience for the UK market. Bored with the small portions and bland taste of the so-called 'healthy options' available, we wanted to create a healthy food offering with lots of choice that didn't compromise on taste or portion size.

Our view is that healthy eating isn't boring. It has nothing to do with sitting in a field nibbling rice cakes and munching sunflower seeds. To us, it is about following a balanced diet that includes lots of fresh fruit and vegetables, some good carbohydrates, loads of water and the odd beer and curry as a reward! It is a philosophical approach to life that means that when you can, you take things easy and in moderation.

You must have respect for your fellow human beings and for your environment, and we are here to help you make these positive changes in your life."

A bit about Vincent the creator (I am a **BIG** fan).

Vincent is a legend – we share a very similar ethos and I love that he is after world domination on the healthy-eating front but also believes in throwing some treats in with the mix (how very SPC!). The winner of numerous food and entrepreneurship awards, he was selected as 'The One to Watch' in the Courvoisier 'The Future 500' announced in January 2008. Vincent also won an Acorn Award in 2009, which is the food industry's leading young person's award with previous winners including Gary Rhodes and Gordon Ramsey. Vincent is a keen supporter of entrepreneurship among young people and is an Ambassador for the Make Your Mark campaign.

My suggestion:
Choose a medium salad base of lettuce leaves.
Then ask for any of the following (depending on how hungry you are):

Protein – chicken breast (farm assured), turkey, bacon, tuna, crayfish, and falafel;

The rest – oven roasted tomatoes, roasted peppers, avocado, hummus, free range egg, broccoli, jalapenos, black olives, tomatoes, cucumber, fresh peppers, mushrooms, red onion, bean sprouts, spring onion, mixed beans, coriander, tomato salsa, and green peas.

Dressing – pick olive oil and lemon, and a nice sprinkling of freshly ground black pepper.
Tossed currently have stores in London but they are going to be rolling out lots more. Yippeeeeeeeee!

For more info go to www.tossed.co.uk

The supermarket sweep

Here are a few suggestions for a quick lunch fix:

Marks and Spencer – grab the following:
- A bag of rocket, spinach and watercress (yum);
- A pack of cooked peeled prawns (sometimes they are 3 for £5);
- An avocado or, if you do not have the facility to chop it up, a pot of guacamole;

I have been known to open the bag of salad, throw in the prawns, a few dollops of guacamole and mix it roughly, and then eat it straight out of the salad bag. The good thing about M&S is near the tills, they have those plastic spoons and forks... perfect for mixing your own salad on the go.

For the veggies:
Sainsbury or Tesco:
- Grab a box of Cauldron marinated (cooked) tofu pieces;
- A small bag of salad;
- A small pot of the best quality hummus you can find;

If you are desperate then also buy a cheap plastic lunch box or food container (you can use it again for a packed lunch). Throw in the tofu pieces on to the salad, half the pot of hummus and enjoy.

Most supermarkets:
- Grab a tin of tuna in sunflower oil (I like the John West No Drain ones);
- A small pot of cottage cheese;
- Bag of salad;

- Small pot of cooked edamame beans
  (often found in the snack section);

Throw it all together for an instant lunch packed full of protein, pulses and lovely salad vitamins. This keeps you going for quite a while!

Snacks on the go

Biltong – one of my favourite snacks on the go. Do not buy the processed one in a packet. Seek out some proper Biltong. I found a place next to a train station the other day. The lovely lady offered to slice me up a fresh one. It was £5 and I divided it up into snacks that kept me going for several days.

If you are in London, there are lots of places that now do 'proper' fresh Biltong in beef, ostrich, springbok and kudu.

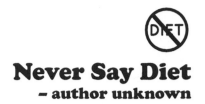

Never Say Diet
– author unknown

"Breakfast
I've weighed my ounce of cereal; the skimmed milk's measured out,
I've performed this ritual many times, so I know what I'm about,
There's tea, no milk, no sugar and half a grapefruit too...
Yes, it's day one of my diet...I've a sense of déjà vu.
By ten o'clock the hunger pangs are getting very strong,
I need a little sustenance to help me get along...
The biscuit tin is beckoning...I need a chocolate fix,
There can't be many calories in this tiny little Twix.

Lunch
I've weighed with great precision two thin slices of brown bread,
And coated them so sparingly with very low-fat spread,
I've got my ounce of cottage cheese, two slices of lean ham,
But I'm dreaming of two doorsteps very thickly spread with jam.
As light snacks go, a sandwich is, of course, quite hard to beat,
But I cannot say that I am feeling that replete.
And then I spot the sweetie jar, just have a little delve,
I check my watch and notice it is twenty-five to twelve...

Tea
I've walked the dog, I've washed the car, I've made the place look neat,
Anything to take my mind off all the food I can't eat,
I've dusted all my ornaments and read the papers...twice.
I'm ready for a cup of tea...with something very nice.
A pack of choc digestives would really fit the bill,
Or three éclairs, or a loaf of bread, or a very large mixed grill.
But it's day one of my diet...and I have to see this through;

Have a stick of celery...and a bag of crisps or two.

Dinner
I've steamed up lots of vegetables to make that slimming soup,
But my mind is in the freezer with that litre of soft scoop.
The slimming magazines all say 'prepare your meals with care',
So I've laid out my two lettuce leaves with quite a lot of flair.
On these I place an appetising skinless chicken breast,
But what would have more appeal is sausage, bacon, egg...
And now that slimmer's pudding...I'll really pig on that...
Kiwi, seedless grapes and yoghurt...yes all of it low-fat.
And so I slowly savour this, my last meal of the day,
Hallucinating all the while of a Chinese Take-Away.
My dreams that night are yes...you guessed...of all forbidden food,
I wake up feeling hungry and in a very sombre mood.
Mount the scales and lo! No change after all that self-control...
Console myself with a Kit-Kat, a bounty and a mini chocolate roll.
And then of course I hate myself, all awash with rage and sorrow,
So I quickly finish off that loaf...and I'll start for real tomorrow!"

Don't count your chickens and other cautionary tales

Here I have outlined a few words of caution, and how you can deal with certain problems. This will really help you if - or when - the particular problem arises.

1. Be careful who you tell

By this, I do not mean that you should keep your SPC lifestyle secret from the world! What I mean is that at the beginning be careful whom you tell. Tell those around you that you know will support you. Remember; in a previous chapter, I gave you a sample letter that you can send to friends and family? It is important that you get the support and belief that you **CAN** change the way you think about food.

One of my clients had experience of this recently. She told her mother-in-law that she was going to be changing the way she thought about food, that she was embarking on a new lifestyle as she was fed up with putting on more and more weight and getting depressed. Her mother-in-law simply said: *"Another diet? You will never stick at it."* This can be a typical response from certain people especially if you have a history of dieting. You can choose to explain to them that you are not doing a quick fix diet. You are changing the way you think about food and intend to use the guidelines for the rest of your life.

If people around you try and sabotage your efforts, then do not discuss it with them anymore. Be the strong one!

2. Be prepared

I cannot stress this point enough, especially at the beginning. Once you are well into the new lifestyle you will find it easy. It takes a while for it to become a habit so have patience and just plan ahead.

I used to get caught out with this repeatedly and now I always carry around emergency options so that I don't get caught out. If you are stuck without anything to eat and you start to get symptoms of low blood sugar, then you will most likely dive into the nearest food place and stuff yourself full of bread/pasta/cakes to satisfy the craving for sugar. If you are anything like me you feel terrible about an hour afterwards... bloated, irritable and still hungry.

I have a small ziplock bag in my handbag (like the ones you take onto an aeroplane with your liquids in). I have a couple of scoops of protein powder in it so that I can easily mix up a protein shake on the go. It helps me instantly and tides me over until I can get into a supermarket and buy something more substantial to eat.

Where possible, plan your day in advance. Know where you are going to be and what food options there will be. This may seem like a chore but at the beginning, it will really help you stay on track. Here is an example of what I mean:

Tomorrow I will be in central London for most of the day:

Wake up at 7.00am

Let dogs out and feed them whilst preparing my breakfast

Eat breakfast 07.30

Walk dogs 08.00

Prepare bag for the day – protein powder in ziplock

First meeting in Baker Street at 09.30, grab a black coffee with splash of cream in Caffe Nero en route

Lunch break scheduled between 12–13.00 – go to Tossed on Baker

Street for lunch

Afternoon meetings scheduled near Waterloo – pick up couple of packs of prawns and cooked chicken in case I finish late. Aim to eat one of them at approx 16.00

Scheduled home time 18.30

Cook dinner at 19.00

Walk dogs 20.00

This all sounds terribly difficult, but I do this mentally before I go to bed at night, it really does help for the following day. It takes me about a minute to think through each evening like this, and I never get caught out without food options. This alone made an enormous difference when I was starting out on my own SPC journey and I take my clients through this process a lot. Start doing it and you will notice a big difference. You can even schedule things in if you have a phone that has a diary or calendar. On the iPhone, I just schedule it in the calendar ie. '16.00hrs have protein shake or chicken breast'. I set an alarm for it and having this regular snack means that I don't get that afternoon slump when I would have satisfied it with some awful refined sugar snack (that often then brought on a headache shortly afterwards!).

3.   Don't keep other food in the fridge.

If you are feeding a family then I can understand that this may be a challenge. **BUT**...if you are struggling with willpower at the beginning, then don't have the sugary stuff visible every time you open the fridge or cupboard. It really won't help. Once you are in the SPC lifestyle, after a few weeks, you will find it much easier. I am just suggesting this to make it all easier from day one. If you have kids, get them to support you in this. Explain what you are doing and that maybe for the first few weeks, you can all have treat day together. I have several clients who have done this and it has not only led to a complete change in eating habits for them, but their children have followed suit and are no longer eating junk.

Another suggestion I have for the first month is that it is better to have treat day away from the house. Not only does it make it more special but also, if you buy in lots of treats and do not eat them all, then you will have to do something with them at the end of treat day. This catches people out sometimes and they end up having 'post treat day breakfast' of cold pizza and chocolate!!!

4. If you have a bad day don't keep it to yourself

You are going to change your life with Six Pack Chick and it is not just a quick weight loss fad. It truly is life changing. New lifestyles take time to get used to and to adapt to. I am not excusing you to have as many slip ups as you want (and go back to old eating habits), but more that I am saying if you **DO** slip up, then don't beat yourself up about it and slump into self-hatred and guilt. Share it! Log on to the Facebook group and share it with other Chicks in the group or on the fan page. You will find plenty of support and most of the people will know exactly how you feel and you can all have a giggle about it. Guilt has no place in your new lifestyle so do not succumb to it.

If you do not have access to Facebook, then try and get an accountability partner who is also doing SPC, and that way you can support each other and give encouragement through any sticky moments.

5. Do not weigh yourself

OK, I know I keep mentioning this but I am going to keep saying it until you get rid of your scales.

I am my smallest size-wise right now and I have absolutely no idea how much I weigh. My strings that I used on day one come out very occasionally now, as I feel so good I don't even need to measure myself. Also, and this is very important...if you are exercising, you will be putting on muscle. Muscle is heavier than fat and therefore by weighing yourself you will not know whether you are putting on muscle or not. You will just become obsessed by the numbers. You will feel so liberated not having to get on them every day and obsessing about the numbers! Please, do it for me :)

6. Do not think you never need another treat day

This happens quite a lot.

I tried not having treat days by way of experiment in the early days. I actually slowed my rate of fat loss right down. What I **DID** do though was think about what I ate on my treat days. When I ate refined sugar in the form of sweets, cakes and chocolate it used to trigger so many of my old health problems that after several months I stopped eating them altogether and just ate fruit and whole grains on my treat day. I felt so much better the day after and I was even more convinced that the headaches and migraines were the result of the sugar. When I don't have refined sugar I don't ever get them.

Really, enjoy your first month of treat days and remember to write everything down on the sheet so that you do not forget to have the foods or drinks that you have thought about during the week. That urge does get less and less as time goes on, and for lots of people, they really do not enjoy the treat days in the way they thought they would. After several months a lot of people just have one 'naughty' on treat day, like a latte with a croissant or a piece of cake for tea.

7. Do not starve yourself

This is very, very, important. This is not a calorie controlled diet and starving yourself long-term will not lead to healthy sustainable fat loss, trust me on this one.

As an experiment, I decided to test the low calorie theory out on myself. I know many of my celebrity clients, who had suffered years of eating very low calorie diets. How hard could it be?

Very!

It really is true that your metabolism slows down. I noticed that for the first couple of weeks I did lose weight (just as much muscle as body fat according to my monitoring system). I felt horrible after a few days; I obsessed about food, dreamed about it, salivated over packets of croissants and just felt miserable.

After a while, I just could not keep it up. You need such huge willpower, and even then, you get to the stage where your body is tired and hungry and you just cannot sustain it any more. That is where the problems begin.

If I tell you that I lost about a stone...and put on a stone and a half. It was like my body had gone into semi-starvation mode and when I started eating 'normally' again my body grabbed on to every single calorie that entered my mouth and deposited it round my middle and around my hips and bottom. It was as if it slapped a load of padding around me in case I ever thought about doing it again.

Because a lot of people have had this calorie counting mentality for a while when they start doing SPC, they apply it to that, too. The good news is that you really don't have to! What a relief, eh? As long as you stick to all the foods that you can eat in abundance and save the other foods for treat day, you can eat away to your heart's content. You will soon discover that you begin to realise what 'true' hunger is. A good friend of mine describes this as the difference between mouth hunger (the hunger that is totally false and usually wants you to eat junk) and true hunger (that stomach growl/ache when it is empty and needs filing again).

You will learn that sense of true hunger again and it is a relief when it finally comes back to you. You stop getting 'mouth hunger' and it feels so liberating. One of my clients said she used to go into supermarkets pre SPC days and spend a good 10 minutes going up that dreadful aisle of pre-packaged cakes. She would be both excited and guilt-ridden at the same time; she would pick out three or four boxes of cakes with the excuse that they would be for her kids after-school treats. Without fail, every time she put her shopping in the car she would munch her way through an entire box of something. The day she did not do it anymore, she rang me up and sobbed down the phone. Now when she goes to the supermarket she does not even bother with that aisle, the kids just enjoy treat day with her. They are healthier and she has dropped three dress sizes.

Losing that last bit if you plateau the 14-day challenge

You will know what I mean when you get to this point and the good news is that you **CAN** shift the last bit. I have designed the 14-day challenge to get rid of that last little bit. If you diarise it then it works! Make yourself accountable to these forms to fill in and go for it.

Reread the plan just to make sure you have not let other foods creep in and really shake up your exercise regime! Try a new exercise a couple of times or schedule in a long walk with a friend... anything to increase the current amount of exercise that you do.

Here is an example of mine:
Day 1: Monday 17th January

Breakfast:	2 poached eggs and 2 slices smoked salmon
Lunch:	Big grilled chicken salad with lentils
Dinner:	Chilli con carne with steamed broccoli
Snacks:	Protein shake at 4pm.
Drinks:	Coffee with breakfast, 4 cups of herbal tea, 1 litre of water
Exercise:	Bikram yoga class (90 minutes), dog walking (90 minutes)

How I felt today: Woke up feeling sluggish but really felt great after yoga, felt totally fired up and ready to lose the last little bit. Needed the protein shake at 4pm. as had a little sweet craving!

Visualisation: Today I visualised that I was walking into a bar to meet a friend, and I was dressed in tight jeans, crisp white shirt and with hair and make-up looking fab. I was confident, smiling and had my head held high.

Six Pack Chick Maintenance

When do you know when you have reached your goal?

I knew I had reached my goal when I felt content. It was a funny moment. I was standing in the changing room of Top Shop with the most awful overhead lighting that in days gone by would have showed up all the dimply thighs and accentuated the curves (where there weren't supposed to be any). I had picked out a pair of jeans. Not super skinny ones – it does not matter how small I could get I just do not have the body type for skinny, low waist jeans.

No, these were slim, straight-legged jeans in white. Yes – white – the very colour of jeans that show up every lump and bump. Sorry I got carried away there...

Anyway, I pulled these jeans up and buttoned them, and noticed there was no muffin top bulging over the top. I turned to the side and really liked what I saw. I was in a pair of size eight white jeans with no muffin top, no lumpy thighs showing through. Really concerned that I might be seeing things I asked the gum-chewing teenage changing room assistant what she thought. She looked me up and down and said: *"They fit you perfectly, they look amazing. You **HAVE** to get them."*

She was not some pushy sales assistant in a designer store earning commission, she couldn't have cared less if I had bought them or not.

Her face was open and genuine.

I bought two pairs.

That is when I knew I had reached my target; I had no idea what I weighed. I threw my scales out a long time ago. The pieces of string, which had given me my progress report for many months, had been sitting in a box unloved for many weeks.

I felt really liberated, my obsession with counting calories had disappeared, and I no longer craved foods constantly. I knew that once a week I could eat what I liked and as long as I stuck to a few simple guidelines, I would be able to sustain it. I sobbed with relief, I really did. Big fat sloppy tears with a smile on my face at the same time. I knew I had to share it with the world, the reason I have written this book for you. You will feel the same way. You can do it!

Starting maintenance

Before you start this phase, you will need new pieces of string. I would suggest buying a different colour string and go through the same measuring process that you did for the initial measuring at the beginning of the book.

Take a photo of yourself, if the budget allows go and get a professional one taken in a piece of clothing you have longed to wear but been unable to get into. If a group of you are doing it then look for a group deal on the internet; you can get some bargain photo shoots done that way. Maintaining the 'new you' is very easy as long as you follow a few simple rules.

Here they are laid out and easy to follow:
You are going to spend the next 4 weeks reintroducing certain foods back into your lifestyle.

So using the original Six Pack Chick foods:

Week 1 - FRUITS

This first week we are going to introduce fruit back into the diet. It is very important that you eat fruit away from other foods at all times. I want you to try and eat fruits with a low Glycaemic Load, as this will prevent spikes in blood sugar after consumption.

A quick explanation of the Glycaemic Index and Glycaemic Load:

Not all carbohydrate foods are created equal; in fact, they behave quite differently in our bodies.

Choosing low GI carbohydrates – the ones that produce only small fluctuations in our blood glucose and insulin levels – is the secret to long-term health reducing your risk of heart disease and diabetes and is the key to sustainable weight loss.

The GI was invented in 1981 by Dr Thomas Wolever and Dr David Jenkins at the University of Toronto, and is a measure of how quickly a food containing 25 or 50 grams of carbohydrate raises blood glucose levels. Because some foods typically have a low carbohydrate content, Harvard researchers created the GL, which takes into account the amount of carbohydrates in a given serving of a food, and so provides a more useful measure. Glycaemic Load also has a scale. Low is 10 or less, medium is 11–19 and 20 or greater is considered high.

Over the page is a list of the Glycaemic Load of various fruits. If there are other fruits that you want to try that aren't on the list, type the name of the fruit into Google to look it up, for example type Glycaemic Load cherries.

Name of Fruit	Serving Size	Glycaemic Load (GL) per serving
Apple	120g	6
Apple Juice (unsweetened)	8 fl oz (250ml)	12
Apricot (dried)	60g	8
Apricot (fresh)	120g	5
Banana	120g	12
Breadfruit	120g	18
Cantaloupe Melon	120g	4
Cherries	120g	3
Cranberry Juice (unsweetened)	8 fl oz (250ml)	16
Dates (dried)	60g	42
Figs (dried)	60g	16
Fruit Salad	120g	9
Grapefruit	120g	3
Grapefruit Juice (unsweetened)	8 fl oz (250ml)	11
Grapes	120g	8
Kiwi	120g	6
Mango	120g	8
Orange	120g	5
Orange Juice (unsweetened)	8 fl oz (250ml)	9
Papaya	120g	10
Peach	120g	5
Peach (canned, natural juice)	120g	4

Name of Fruit	Serving Size	Glycaemic Load (GL) per serving
Pear	120g	4
Pears (canned, natural juice)	120g	5
Pineapple	120g	7
Pineapple Juice (unsweetened)	8 fl oz (250ml)	16
Plantain (boiled)	120g	8
Plums	120g	5
Prunes	60g	10
Raisins	60g	28
Strawberries	120g	1
Tomato Juice	8 fl oz (250ml)	4
Watermelon	120g	4

As you can see, some dried fruits gave a much higher load than fresh so should be avoided. Fruit juice does, too, because it does not have the fibre in it. I would much rather you had the whole fruit than a glass of fruit juice so please avoid them.

So, for this first week you are going to stay with the SPC foods and have one piece of fruit in the morning and one in the afternoon, six days a week, and then you are going to have your treat day just as you did before.

Week 2 – NUTS AND SEEDS

In Week 2 you are going to be introducing nuts and seeds back into the diet; use them as a mid morning or mid afternoon snack. Nuts and seeds have different nutrient profiles so here is a little information on them; I have listed them in order of preference on the SPC method:

Mixed nuts

Often I buy big bags of lots of different nuts and mix them all up in an airtight container. I then dispense them into mini snack pots and carry them around with me. **WORD OF WARNING:** If nuts are big 'cascade' foods for you then approach with caution. They are very high in calories and whilst a small handful makes a good snack, that is all it can be ...no reaching into the pot for seconds and thirds.

Buy your nuts from somewhere where you know they are going to have a high turnover of stock; some nuts can have fungal problems if sat in a warm, damp storeroom for a period of time.

I order mine online from Julian Graves, www.juliangraves.com and have found them to be good quality.

Almonds: Almonds are high in vitamin E and have more magnesium than most nuts. A quarter cup of whole almonds (about the same as a 1 oz. serving size), has nearly the amount of calcium as a quarter cup of milk.

Nutrition per ounce:
- Calories: 160;
- Fat: 14 grams (1 saturated (s), 9 monounsaturated (m), 3 polyunsaturated (p));
- Protein: 6 grams;
- Other notable nutrients: Over 35% of your daily requirement of vitamin E, over 30% for manganese, and almost 20% for riboflavin and magnesium.

Walnuts: Walnuts are the only nut with alpha-linolenic acid, an omega-3 fatty acid. They also have vitamin E and magnesium.

Nutrition per ounce:
- Calories: 190;
- Fat: 18 grams (1.5 s, 2.5 m, 13 p);
- Protein: 4 grams;
- Other notable nutrients: The World's Healthiest Foods reports that walnuts have special anti-inflammatory benefits because they contain tannins, tellimagrandin, the flavonol morin, and quinone juglone (which are found in almost no other food).

Peanuts: Peanuts (technically legumes) have the most folate of any nuts.

Nutrition per ounce:
- Calories: 170;
- Fat: 14 grams (2 s, 7 m, 4 p);
- Protein: 7 grams;
- Other notable nutrients: Almost 20% of your daily value of niacin and 10% of folate and vitamin E.

Cashews: Cashews have more magnesium than almonds. Most of the unsaturated fat in cashews is oleic acid, which is the same fat that is in heart-healthy olive oil.

Nutrition per ounce:
- Calories: 160;
- Fat: 13 grams (3 s, 8 m, 2 p);
- Protein: 4 grams;
- Other notable nutrients: Cashews contain over 5% of the recommended daily values of vitamin K and iron.

The Least-healthy nuts

There is no 'worst nut'. Anything is bad for you when you over-indulge – but macadamia nuts and pecans are to watch out for because they are higher in calories than other nuts. While they are only about 10 calories per serving higher than some of the other nuts listed above, they are also higher in fat and lower in protein. Ounce for ounce, they just aren't quite as good as some of the others.

Macadamia Nuts

Nutrition per ounce:

- Calories: 200;
- Fat: 22 grams (3.5 s, 17 m, .5 p);
- Protein: 2 grams;
- Other notable nutrients: A 1 oz. serving contains 6% of the daily recommended value of iron and over 20% of the recommended value of thiamine.

Pecans

Nutrition per ounce:

- Calories: 200;
- Fat: 20 grams (2 s, 12 m, 6 p);
- Protein: 3 grams;
- Other notable nutrients: A 1 oz. serving of pecans contains 8% of the recommended daily value of thiamine and 16% of the recommend daily value of copper.

Interestingly enough, pecans and macadamia nuts, which are both high in calories and fat (and some of the tastiest nuts in my opinion), are also the most expensive nuts.

Seeds are another great snack that we are introducing back into the mix.

Pumpkin seeds in particular are a great addition back into the SPC lifestyle. They have been linked to various medicinal claims and eating them can only do you good! They are high in manganese, magnesium, phosphorus, tryptophan, iron, copper, vitamin K, zinc, protein and, along with sunflower seeds, are high in phytosterols. Phytosterols are compounds found in plants that have a chemical structure very similar to cholesterol, and when present in the diet in sufficient amounts, are believed to reduce blood levels of cholesterol, enhance the immune response and decrease risk of certain cancers.

Sunflower seeds are an excellent source of vitamin E, the body's primary fat-soluble antioxidant. Vitamin E travels throughout the body neutralizing free radicals that would otherwise damage fat-containing structures and molecules, such as cell membranes, brain cells, and cholesterol. By protecting these cellular and molecular components, vitamin E has significant anti-inflammatory effects that result in the reduction of symptoms in asthma, osteoarthritis, and rheumatoid arthritis, conditions where free radicals and inflammation play a big role. Vitamin E has also been shown to reduce the risk of colon cancer, help decrease the severity and frequency of hot flushes in women going through menopause, and help reduce the development of diabetic complications.

Sunflower seeds are also high in vitamin B1, manganese, magnesium, copper, tryptophan, selenium, phosphorus, vitamin B5 and folate. Gandhi once observed, *"Wherever flaxseed becomes a regular food item among people, there will be better health."* The warm, earthy and subtly nutty flavour of flaxseeds, combined with an abundance of omega-3 fatty acids, makes them an increasingly popular addition to the diet of many a health conscious consumer. Whole and ground flaxseeds, as well as flaxseed oil, are available throughout the year.

Flaxseeds are slightly larger than sesame seeds and have a hard shell that is smooth and shiny. Their colour ranges from deep amber to reddish brown depending upon whether the flax is of the golden or brown variety. While whole flaxseeds feature a soft crunch, the nutrients in ground seeds are more easily absorbed. Flaxseeds and flaxseed oil are popular among vegans and vegetarians who want a non-animal source of omega-3 fatty acids. Apart from omega-3 fatty acids, flaxseeds are high in manganese, fibre, magnesium, folate, copper, phosphorus, and vitamin B6.

Here are some suggestions for adding seeds to your diet:
- Add sunflower seeds to your favourite tuna, chicken or turkey salad recipe.
- Garnish mixed green salads with sunflower seeds.
- Adding sunflower seeds to scrambled eggs will give them a unique taste and texture.
- Use fine ground sunflower seeds to dust your meats with in place of flour.
- Add pumpkin seeds to healthy sautéed vegetables.
- Sprinkle pumpkin seeds on top of mixed green salads.
- Grind pumpkin seeds with fresh garlic, parsley and coriander leaves. Mix with olive oil and lemon juice for a tasty salad dressing.
- Next time you make burgers, whether it be from vegetables, turkey or beef, add some ground pumpkin seeds.
- To pump up the nutritional volume of your protein shake, add ground flaxseeds before blending.
- To give cooked vegetables a nuttier flavour, sprinkle some ground flaxseeds on top of them.

Week 3 – GRAINS

Grains...hmmmm...tricky.

A lot of you will probably have scanned through this book on the day you bought it looking to see whether you could ever have bread and pasta again.

(Bridget pauses and smiles...)
I would have done exactly the same thing a few years ago.

Personally, I eat very few grains. If I am doing a lot of exercise and need the added complex carbohydrate then I consume them, but apart from that, I don't.

In my case, I could not stop eating them before. I could not just pick up one slice of baguette and nibble on it; I would eat the whole loaf. My brain saw it as exactly the same as a bag of sweets and I would have no cut off point.

For some people it is not realistic never to eat any grains again, but I would request that you only eat wholegrains to include the following:
- Brown rice;
- Barley;
- Quinoa (pronounced keen-wa);
- Spelt;
- Wholemeal pasta;
- Rye bread;
- Whole oats.

Please do not start down the *'I will just have one piece of processed white toast'* road. It offers absolutely no nutritional benefit whatsoever, it spikes blood sugar and leaves you craving more sugar...trust me!

I recommend that if you are to eat grains, then you eat them pre-exercise. Only have a portion the same size as a balled fist (yours, not Mike Tyson's).

Stick to no more than one portion on an exercise day...

You can eat with all the recommendations in this book for **THE REST OF YOUR LIFE**. It is so easy.

If you get out of control again for whatever reason, just do two weeks of strict following, as if you were on day one again. You will refocus and your cravings will disappear again.

I have been eating like this for a long time and I have never been healthier; my immune system is strong, my skin is clear and glowing, my hair is thick and long and my mood is happy pretty much all of the time.

Exercise – just in case you thought, I had forgotten all about it

I am only writing one page about exercise.
Yes; you read that correctly.

I have had many Personal Training clients and I love it when clients who walked in to the first session saying, "I hate exercise", leave with a big smile on their face.

Although nowadays I still see clients for training, I spend more of my time overseeing the Six Pack Chick one-day events and looking after all the people in the group.

Exercise is very important to me; I love it. I do not enjoy **ALL** forms of exercise though and I believe very strongly in finding the exercise **YOU** love.

One of London's top Personal Trainers is the wonderful Jean-Pierre de Villiers. I am very lucky to have him as my trainer. Why do I need a trainer? I believe that you always learn more, even when highly qualified, and I work much harder in his sessions than I would on my own. He is a legend and he has joined Six Pack Chick as the fitness guru.

I asked him to write about exercise in my book; he is a great motivator and here is an extract from his book, *77 Ways to Reshape Your Life*.

MOVE
It may not feel like it during your first few training sessions, but your body is designed to move! These days we are more sedentary than

ever and the detrimental effects of this are becoming increasingly apparent throughout society, from postural problems to weight gain and depression.

The more active you can be every day the greater benefits you will see in how you look and feel. These benefits go beyond reducing fat and include improved mobility, flexibility, mood, energy levels and all the wonderful life-changing benefits that these improvements bring.

We constantly rely on machines to do things for us and to get us from A to B, but your body is a machine as well, and for too many people it is being left to deteriorate through neglect. Walk, cycle, swim, run, **MOVE**.

Get active every day of your life, at every opportunity and in every way imaginable and begin to appreciate your body for the amazing piece of engineering that it is.

JP and I often think up ways to make exercise more fun for our clients. We both believe that if you can laugh with your clients, especially when working them really hard, it makes it so much more fun. Laughter is the only way I can get through some of my workouts! Here JP talks about perception:

"Making exercise enjoyable is an important factor that is often overlooked. People go to the gym or start doing exercise because they want to be healthier, lose weight and get fit. But most people give up after just a few months, weeks, or sometimes even days. Because they have the perception of exercise being boring and painful, it is the last thing that they actually want to do when they wake up in the morning or have just finished work.

Why would you go somewhere you don't want to be? You'd rather be at home or with friends or out for drinks or watching a movie...doing something enjoyable, right? What most people don't realise is that to reshape their bodies and, if they let it, their lives, they need to start by changing their perception of exercise."

Often on my blog I talk about exercise classes that I have tried. I love finding classes that leave women smiling, confident and counting down the days until the next one. From Zumba to in-line skating, from Pilates to pole dancing, there IS an exercise out there that **YOU** will **LOVE**.

Check out my blog www.bridgethunt.com

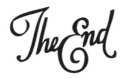

This is not the end only the beginning

Thank you for reading... *Mother Hen*

Candida Questionnaire

This questionnaire is designed for adults and the scoring system is not appropriate for children. It lists factors in your medical history, which promote the growth of Candida Albicans (Section A), and symptoms commonly found in individuals with yeast-connected illness (Sections B and C).

For each 'Yes' answer in Section A, circle the point score in that section. Total your score and record it on the line at the end of the section. Then move on to Sections B and C and score as directed.

Filling out and scoring this questionnaire should help you evaluate the possible role of candida in contributing to your health problem. They will not provide an automatic 'Yes' or 'No' answer.

If you would like more information on testing for Candida, please visit the website of Genova Diagnostics: www.gdx.uk.net
or call them on: +44 (0)20 8336 7750

Please turn the page to begin.

Section A

Q.		Pts.
1.	Have you taken tetracyclines (or other antibiotics) for 2 months (or longer)?	25
2.	Have you, at any time in your life, taken other 'broad spectrum' antibiotics (including Keflex®, ampicillin, amoxicillin, Ceclor®, Bactrim®, and Septra®*) for respiratory, urinary or other infections (for 2 months or longer, or in shorter courses 4 or more times in a 1-year period)?	20
3.	Have you, at any time in your life, been troubled by persistent vaginal problems or had 3 or more episodes of vaginitis in a year?	25
4.	Have you been pregnant 2 or more times? Have you been pregnant once?	5 3
5.	Have you taken birth control pills for more than 2 years? For 6 months to 2 years?	15 8
6.	Have you taken prednisone, Decadron® or other cortisone-type drugs for more than 2 weeks? For 2 weeks or less?	15 6
7.	Does exposure to perfumes, insecticides, fabric shop odours and other chemicals provoke: Moderate to severe symptoms? Mild symptoms?	 20 5
8.	Are your symptoms worse on damp, muggy days or in mouldy places?	20
9.	Have you had persistent athlete's foot, 'jock itch', or other chronic fungus infections of the skin or nails? Have such infections been... Severe or persistent? Mild to moderate?	 20 10

Q.		Pts.
10.	Do you crave sugar?	10
11.	Do you crave breads?	10
12.	Do you crave alcoholic beverages?	10
13.	Does tobacco smoke really bother you?	10

TOTAL SCORE, Section A

* Such antibiotics kill off 'good germs' while they're killing off those which cause infection.

Section B: Major Symptoms

For each symptom which is present, enter the appropriate figure in the point score column:

If a symptom is **mild**, score 3 points.

If a symptom is **moderate**, score 6 points.

If a symptom is **severe** or **disabling**, score 9 points.

Add total score for this section and record it on the line at the end of this section.

Section B

Q.	Symptom	Pts.
1.	Fatigue or lethargy.	
2.	Feeling of being 'drained'	
3.	Poor memory	
4.	Feeling 'spacey' or 'unreal'	

Q.	Symptom	Pts.
5.	Depression	
6.	Numbness, burning or tingling	
7.	Muscle aches	
8.	Muscle weakness or paralysis	
9.	Pain and/or swelling in joints	
10.	Abdominal pain	
11.	Constipation	
12.	Diarrhoea	
13.	Bloating	
14.	Troublesome vaginal discharge	
15.	Persistent vaginal burning or itching	
16.	Prostatitis	
17.	Impotence	
18.	Loss of sexual feeling	
19.	Endometriosis	
20.	Dysmenorrhoea	
21.	Premenstrual tension	
22.	Spots in front of eyes	
23	Erratic vision	

TOTAL SCORE, Section B

Section C: Other Symptoms

For each symptom which is present, enter the appropriate figure in the point score column:

If a symptom is **mild**, score 1 point.

If a symptom is **moderate**, score 2 points.
If a symptom is **severe** or **disabling**, score 3 points.

Add total score for this section and record it on the line at the end of this section.

* While the symptoms in this section occur commonly in patients with yeast-connected illness, they also occur commonly in patients who do not have candida.

Section C

Q.	Symptom	Pts.
1.	Drowsiness	
2.	Irritability or jitteriness	
3.	Incoordination	
4.	Inability to concentrate	
5.	Frequent mood swings	
6.	Headache	
7.	Dizziness / loss of balance	
8.	Pressure above ears… feeling of head swelling and tingling	
9.	Itching	
10.	Other rashes	
11.	Heartburn	
12.	Indigestion	
13.	Belching and intestinal gas	
14.	Mucus in stools	
15.	Haemorrhoids	

Q.	Symptom	Pts.
16.	Dry mouth	
17.	Rash or blisters in mouth	
18.	Bad breath	
19.	Joint swelling or arthritis	
20.	Nasal congestion or discharge	
21.	Postnasal drip	
22.	Nasal itching	
23.	Sore or dry throat	
24.	Cough	
25.	Pain or tightness in chest	
26.	Wheezing or shortness of breath	
27.	Urgency or urinary frequency	
28.	Burning on urination	
29.	Failing vision	
30.	Burning or tearing eyes	
31.	Recurrent ear infections	
32.	Fluid in ears	
33.	Ear pain or deafness	
34.	Tubes in ears	
35.	Other symptoms:	

TOTAL SCORE, Section C

GRAND TOTAL SCORE
(Add up Total Score for Sections A, B, and C)

Evaluation:

(Note that the scoring will be different for females and males since seven questions apply exclusively to women, while only two apply exclusively to men.)

If your point score is over **180 in women** (and **140 in men**), Candida almost certainly plays a role in causing your health problems.

If your point score is **over 120 in women** (and **90 in men**), Candida probably plays a role in causing your health problems.

If your point score is **60 to 120 for women** (and **40 to 90 in men**), Candida possibly plays a role in causing your health problems.

If your point score is **less than 60 for women** (and **40 for men**), Candida is less apt to be playing a significant role in causing your health problems.

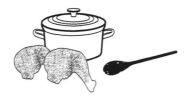

Recipes

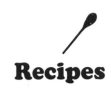

Recipes

Some of the recipes in this section are my own and some of them are from the fabulous Chicks and Chaps who are clients or members of my secret Facebook group. I will be releasing a recipe book but in the meantime, here are a selection of some of my favourite recipes.

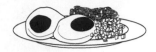

The Ultimate SPC Breakfast

(by Huevos Rancheros, Serves 1)

In search of the ultimate SPC breakfast, I tried making this one morning. It kept me full until about 2pm. So delicious!!!

Ingredients

Two of the freshest omega-3-rich eggs or Burford Browns;

1/2 can black beans, drained and mashed;

1 tablespoon of extra virgin olive oil or a generous teaspoon of coconut oil (for a different taste);

1 teapoon lemon juice;

sea salt and pepper, to taste;

tablespoon of home-made tomato salsa (see next recipe p160);

1/4 avocado, sliced; chopped coriander (optional);

a pinch of cayenne pepper.

Poach eggs (see right).

Method

Heat beans in a frying pan while eggs are cooking. Remove beans from heat and mix in olive oil, lemon juice, salt and pepper. Add a pinch of cayenne for spicy beans. Place beans on plate, top with poached eggs, avocado, salsa and coriander.

Recipes

The perfect poached egg

The perfect poached egg is something of a personal obsession. I have tried every method out there and merit goes to Delia Smith's shallow frying pan method and Hugh Fearnley-Whittingstall's 'vortex' method, but the following method is perfect if you are struggling for time and don't want messy washing up!

If you are going to poach an egg, and do not want to spend 20 minutes cleaning the pan; here is what to do:

- Buy some microwaveable cling film;
- Get a cup or a small ramekin;
- Push the cling film into the cup/ramekin, and crack the egg into the cling film;
- You should be able to tie the cling film around the top of the egg;
- Drop egg into boiling water, and poach.

Fabulous.

Sexy Smoking Salsa

(by Peter Merrens)

Peter is a fabulous cook; he has cooked for me many times and really should be a chef. His knowledge of herbs, spices and creating healthy dishes is second to none. Here are a few of his best recipes!!!

For a large bowl of salsa:
The best salsa tomatoes smell deeply of tomato stalks and are red all the way through. You can make salsa from fully green tomatillos but we rarely see them in the UK. So good toms = good salsa. Coriander goes off within a day. I stay away from fresh chillies, as they can be a little uncontrollable because they vary in heat so much. The white balsamic vinegar is for sweetness and works with tomatoes. One could use Agave syrup but it would be frowned on by, shhh, you know who...

Ingredients

- 2 packs of small (say) Sultan's Jewel tomatoes;
- 1/2 super sweet onion;
- 1 small bunch of fresh coriander;
- 2 teaspoons of white balsamic vinegar;
- 1 dessertspoon olive oil;
- 1/2 teaspoon chipotle chilli paste or powder;
- 1 teaspoon sweet smoked paprika;
- 1 large grated clove of garlic;
- Pinch of sea salt;
- 1/2 fresh lime;
- A food processor with a blade.
- Prep (5 minutes max)

Method

Rinse tomatoes. Wash the onion and cut it up a little to give it a head start. Put all the ingredients **EXCEPT** the lime and the salt in the processor and whizz until salsa consistency.

Use a rough cut for tuna, etc., and a finer consistency for dipping.

When it is done, add the lime juice, to give it any desired tang.

Then, and if you must, add a pinch of salt.

The salsa will separate in the bowl after a while so just stir the water from the tomatoes back in when needed.

It will keep in the fridge overnight to have with eggs in the morning but not any longer than that... **enjoy!**

Asparagus, smoked ham, red pepper and cottage cheese tortilla.

(For a 4-person tortilla. or one person for 4 meals!)
Total prep time about 20 minutes.

Try to have almost the same amount of vegetables as eggs. The trick with this omelette is to nurse it whilst it is cooking. Our Iberian cousins put it in the oven but it makes for a much heavier affair than the holiday fling it should be.

Ingredients

300g of asparagus tips;
8 Piquillo peppers (from a jar are pricey but vital unless you want to grill and peel your own peppers);
2 tablespoons cottage cheese (any);

Small bag of fresh flat leaf parsley;
Small bunch of fresh chives;
Dried chilli flakes (any);
Olive oil for frying;
100 g cooked smoked ham;

8 large fresh eggs (fresh as possible);
A few twists of black pepper;
A dessert spoon of salt (just to cook the asparagus).

Method

Prep: Turn on the oven to 180°c. Boil some water with all the salt and get the asparagus on straight away. Cook it until tender then rinse off the salt in cold water and chop them into inch lengths. Beat the eggs so that they are foamy on top. (This lightness transfers to the omelette.) Take the Piquillo peppers (I saw them in Sainsbury's this morning so I know they are around) out of the jar and pat them free of oil. Slice them into thin strips and combine with the asparagus. Slice up the ham in the same way. Get two tablespoons of cottage cheese ready. Rough chop two handfuls of parsley. Fine chop a small handful of chives.

Cook: Heat 2 tablespoons of olive oil in the pan over a medium heat. Fold the coolish asparagus, the ham, a pinch of chilli, almost all the parsley, all the chives, the peppers and the cottage cheese into the beaten eggs. The ingredients will clump together so make sure you spread them out. When the oil is hot, put in all the egg mixture. Proportion the vegetables around the pan. Whilst cooking, ease up the sides of the tortilla and tip up the omelette to let the egg mixture get to the frying pan surface a few times. You should be trying to slightly drain off the top of the omelette. When it still looks damp on top but it is not swimming and the tortilla is lightly brown on the bottom, take the pan and shove it in the oven. The beaten egg and cottage cheese might make the top a little light and puffy. This is not traditional but it sure is fun. When it is a nice brown around the edges on top of the omelette, take it out for a second. Test it with a knife blade to make sure that by coming out clean, it is cooked in the middle. You can swap it between the hob and the oven a few times but be careful if you have heated up the handle. Let it cool a bit, give it a sprinkle of parsley and slice it up!

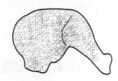

Hungarian Paprika Chicken

(another Peter Merrens special, for 2 or 3)

I used to be married to a Hungarian woman who, bless, could not really cook, neither could her Mum. They made this dish for me once and it was terrible. Then, when visiting their family in Budapest, I had it again and it was to die for. The difference was that her Mum was mean with the paprika. Go figure.

This dish is an easy to make traditional Hungarian chicken casserole. It works for us as it has no wine or root vegetables. It can be refrigerated or frozen and reheated as long as you heat it thoroughly. Chicken thighs are best in all casseroles as they do not dry out in the same way as a chicken breast. Serve it with cauliflower mash or courgette strips and a mound of salad.

Ingredients

(A deep frying pan with a lid is required)

6 skinless and boneless chicken thighs (get free-range, corn fed if you can);

3 heaped tablespoons of sweet paprika;

1 dessertspoon of cumin seeds;

3 garlic cloves;

1 medium red onion;

6 Romano red peppers (long thin ones);

1 lemon;

A pinch of sea salt;

Olive oil for cooking;

A few sprigs of coriander;

Method

Prep

Put a mix of the spices into a small dish.

De-seed and cut the peppers into skinny fries.

Dice the onion.

Rough chop the garlic.

Dry off the chicken thighs and cut off any tendons showing.

Cook

Heat up the oil and brown each thigh nicely all over. Remove them from the pan. Add the onion to the pan and fry until going transparent than chuck in the garlic and fry both until they begin to colour. Put the paprika and cumin in the pan and mix together the spices with the onions and oil. Fry for another 20 seconds, stirring so the spices do not burn then add the chicken and coat it all over in the mix. Then add the peppers to the pan. (There will seem to be too many peppers ...have no fear, they will break down.) Give it all a stir to mix it up, and then add no more than 3 tablespoons of water to the pan. Put on the lid, turn down the heat to a simmer and cook it for about an hour to an hour and a half, stirring every 10 minutes to stop the bottom burning. It will be ready when the chicken flakes away with a fork and the peppers should be recognisable but completely soft. The peppers will have added their juices to the dish. If there is too much juice in the pan at the end, I take out the ingredients leaving the juices and rapidly boil the juices to thicken then add it all back together. Just before serving, taste once again. If a little too rich, one brief squeeze of lemon will help. Serve with some coriander leaves on top. The Hungarians serve it with sour cream... why not try it with a little cottage cheese to see if it works?

Curry pork burgers with spicy lentils and spinach

Ingredients

500g lean pork mince;
1 red onion, grated;

2 tablespoon tandoori curry paste;

A small bunch coriander;
1 egg.

Method

Put the mince, onion, curry paste and half the coriander in a bowl, season and mix really well. Form into 4 burgers (You can freeze at this stage if you want to).

Char grill for about 4–5 minutes each side until cooked through. Serve with finely shredded white cabbage in a dressing of oil, lemon juice, salt and pepper and a dash of wholegrain mustard.

Or... as recommended... serve with:

Spicy lentils

(I like to make a big pot of this)

Ingredients

250g red lentils;
1 tablespoon coconut
  oil
1 garlic clove, crushed;

Fingertip piece fresh
  root ginger, grated;
2 teapoon garam
  masala;

100g baby spinach
  leaves; I like frozen
  ones;
Few coriander leaves;

Method

Boil lentils for 8–12 minutes, then drain. Meanwhile, heat the oil in a pan and gently cook the garlic, ginger and garam masala for 2–3 minutes.

Mix this with the drained lentils and warm through.

Serve a big dollop of lentils on the plate and put pork burger on top. This is a complete Six Pack Chick meal - protein, pulses and vegetables.

SPC Tuscan Sausage Stew

(adapted from Fay's Family Food by Fay Ripley) – Joan Cornally

Joan is one of my all time favourite clients. Joan and I share a very similar addiction to sugar and I learnt a huge amount about myself in my one-to-one sessions with her. Joan is an exceptional nanny (she is the ultimate Supernanny) and she has a love of Italy and travelling. Her cooking is fabulous and I am glad one of her recipes is here.

Ingredients

6 Debbie and Andrew's sausages;

1 table spoon olive oil or a little coconut oil;

1 med onion;

1 celery stick;

1 med red pepper;

1 organic chicken stock cube;

2 tins tomatoes;

1 tin cannellini beans (drained and rinsed);

1 tablespoon tomato puree;

1 bay leaf;

1 teaspoon dried oregano.

Method

Pre Heat oven to 180°c (fan), 200°c or gas mark 6.

Brown sausages in a casserole dish in the oil for 5 minutes, and then cut each sausage in 4.

When they are well on their way, add the chopped onion, celery and pepper to soften.

Add a little more oil if needed and cook for 10 more minutes.

Dissolve the stock cube in just a mug of boiling water and add to the pot along with the tinned tomatoes, cannellini beans, tomato puree, bay leaf and oregano.

Bring to simmering point and cover.

Cook in the oven with the lid on for 30–40 minutes.

You can serve it with a light salad, chickpea spaghetti or a dish of green veg.

You can also add lentils whilst cooking to give this extra bulk.

(Slow cooked) Beef, lentil and vegetable soup

(by Loreen Gaye)

I first met Loreen through teaching Zumba and she very quickly became a fabulous member of Six Pack Chicks. Loreen is one of the most positive people I have ever met. She approaches life with the biggest smile on her face and is the most wonderful inspiration to new members of the group. Loreen has invented many recipes for her slow cooker, and is the SPC slow cooking **EXPERT***!*

Ingredients

(Slow Cooker and Frying Pan required)

500g lean stewing beef;
1 cup red of lentil beans;
2/3 cloves of garlic – diced;
2 stalks of spring onions – chopped;
¼ red, yellow and green peppers – diced;

1 leek – thinly sliced;
1 small courgette – diced;
1 cup of marrow – diced;
1 cup of shredded cabbage;
1 teaspoon dried mixed herbs;

1 teaspoon dried herbs de Provence;
Pinch of course black pepper;
Pinch of sea salt;
Virgin olive oil;
2 Kallo stock cubes (beef).

Method

Heat slow cooker on High for half an hour before use.
Add oil to pan. Sauté onions, garlic, spring onions and peppers until soften then add to slow cooker. Add leeks, courgette and

Recipes

shredded cabbage and marrow to pan heat through then add to slow cooker. If required add more oil to pan then add stewing beef, season with dried herbs, salt and pepper. Brown off meat then add to slow cooker.

Prepare beef stock as directed on packet add to slow cooker.

Wash lentils and add to slow cooker.

Cook on **LOW** for 8 hours.

Note: Usually done overnight or first thing in the morning, so ready when I come home from work.

Savoury courgette loaf

(by Mei Tse)

Mei is one of life's treasures. She is a keen little baker and has designed this SPC friendly 'bread'. Here is her version of a Savoury Courgette Loaf. **Absolutely delicious.**

Ingredients

- 1 large grated courgette;
- 1 medium onion, grated;
- 1/3 cup of extra virgin olive oil;
- 2 eggs;
- 3 cups gram flour;
- 1 1/2 teaspoons baking soda;
- 1/2 teaspoon baking powder;
- 1/2 teaspoon salt.

Method

Preheat oven to Gas mark 4. Grease a loaf pan. In a bowl, mix together grated courgette, onion, eggs and olive oil. In a separate bowl, mix together flour, salt, baking soda and baking powder. Fold the wet ingredients into the dry. Pour the batter into the pan and bake for about 30 minutes, **OR** until you stick a knife into the centre and it comes out clean. Let it cool down, and then enjoy your SPC friendly loaf.

Mei's thoughts: *"It turned out quite well; I treated it like toast accompanying my chicken salad. It is the first time I have used gram flour and I found it is quite strong in flavour so it did not taste like how I expected it to. Still, I enjoyed it and cannot wait to experiment more with it."*

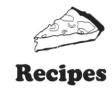

Recipes

Giant onion flan

(by Leah Hearle)

I think Leah is not only the best osteopath in the world, but she is also a fabulous cook. Her constant smiling face and creativity in the kitchen make her such wonderful company!

"This is like a giant red onion pancake. It is great for a packed lunch and can be cut up into slices, and kept in the fridge for a week. I was given the recipe by a lady in the local health food shop. Here goes...roughly:"

Method

Cut red onions into slices, add herbs (I used whatever was in the garden... rosemary, thyme, parsley) and season with sea salt and freshly ground pepper. Cover generously in olive oil.

In another bowl, make a batter with gram of flour and water.

A nice seasoning for the batter is cumin, coriander seeds and salt and pepper.

Add the onions to the batter and place straight on to tray and in the oven until brown.

This took about 40 minutes on the top shelf of the Aga.

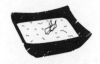

The best ever Dhal recipe

(by Afia Yasin)

I will never forget the first time Afia cooked for me. She even sent me home with food parcels. The best Asian cooking in the world. I want her to open a restaurant called Simply Afia.

I will try and help but having never followed any recipes for south Asian food it could be tricky. I will try and give you measurements, however, please experiment.

Ingredients

2 cups dhal;
1 onion (white/red or handful of spring);
a few garlic cloves;
ghee or oil.

Depending on the dhal and individual taste, you will need the following spices:

Salt, chilli and turmeric;
Chat masala *(this is my personal addition because I like sour things);*
Cumin seeds and maybe garam masala.

Method

First, you wash and soak the dhal; the longer the better. Cook the dhal with 1 teaspoon of salt, 1 teaspoon of chilli and 1/4 teaspoon of turmeric, 1/2 teaspoon of ground cumin and ground coriander seeds and, if you like, a teaspoon of chat masala and garlic cloves. Adjust this after tasting, with more chilli or salt.

Bring the dhal to boil and keep adding boiling water until the dhal and spices meld and become one and the consistency is soupy but **NOT** watery.

You then fry an onion (white, red or spring) in ghee, oil or whatever you want, and once the onions soften, add cumin seeds.

(When the onion and cumin turn slightly brown.) Pour this over the dhal and add fresh chopped coriander. If the dhal is chunky, then you can add a sprinkling of garam masala.

Hope this helps everyone.

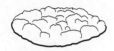

Spicy gram flour flatbreads

(by Helen English)

I know Helen through dancing; she looks like one of the Nolan Sisters. She has a wicked sense of humour and really is one of life's smilers. She is also a fantastic cook; she came up with these flatbreads and they are divine. Sometimes I eat one with a poached egg on top for breakfast. **Yum.**

Ingredients

200g gram flour;
220ml water;
Pinch of salt;

1/2 teapoon each of
turmeric, ground
cumin, ground
coriander, paprika

and cayenne pepper
and a little chopped
coriander.

Method

Whizz it all up and leave it to rest for 10 minutes.

Fry like pancakes in coconut oil. Serve with whatever you like; I did some seared steak in Indian spices with onions, garlic and ginger and a side salad.

Oh, and the quantities made 5 side-plate sized flatbreads.

Diet? What diet?

Egg and cottage cheese breakfast muffins

(by Sanaria Baban)

I have never met Sanaria face to face but I cannot wait for the day I meet her. She is the wife of a friend of mine and is clearly a major talent in the kitchen. She posted this recipe up in the Facebook group to great applause and excitement!

Ingredients

1 cup cottage cheese;
4 eggs (lightly beaten);
1 cup gram flour;
1 teaspoon baking powder;

1/4 teaspoon salt;
1/4 cup chicken breast (or any meat that you like) chopped;

2 green onions (sliced);
oil.

Method

Mix the cottage cheese, eggs, flour, baking powder and salt in a bowl. Stir in the chicken and green onions.
Rub some oil in the baking dish to prevent sticking.

Bake in a preheated 200°C oven until they are golden brown on top and a toothpick poked into the centre comes out clean; about 25–30 minutes.

Warm chicken salad with summer vegetables and chickpeas for two

(Another Leah Hearle special)

Ingredients

Olive oil;

2 chicken breasts (sliced);

1 red onion (sliced);

1 small garlic clove (sliced very fine);

1/2 lemon;

Heaped teaspoon paprika;

1 red pepper (cubes);

1 courgette (cubes);

Can of chickpeas;

Bunch of fresh basil chopped;

A couple handfuls of spinach;

Salt and pepper.

Method

Heat pan then add a dash of oil and the sliced onions and fry in non-stick frying pan (uses less oil). Begin to brown then add garlic immediately, followed by chicken.

When it is all sealed and begins to brown, add paprika; it gets a little dry so it is a good point to squeeze in some lemon juice and season to taste.

Turn down the heat a notch and add the courgettes and peppers. Then add chickpeas.

Cook out for a few minutes before taking off the heat and stirring in basil.

Dress the spinach on a large plate with salt and pepper, lemon juice and olive oil.

Put the hot chicken on top.

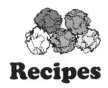

Recipes

Falafels

(by Helen English, *Helen, please move into my house...!*)

Ingredients

1 tin of chickpeas;
1/2 onion;
1 large clove of garlic;
Fresh coriander;
Fresh parsley;

2 pinches of cumin powder;
2 pinches of ground coriander;
1 pinch of cayenne pepper;

2 dessert spoons of gram flour (available in most supermarkets and Asian food shops).

Method

Blend them all together until they form a thick sticky dough ball.

Form into patties.

Dust lightly with more gram flour. Press in some sesame seeds for extra crunch.

Usually they would then be deep-fried but I tried shallow frying them in coconut oil until lightly golden, and then finish them in the oven on a medium heat for 15–20 minutes.

For the sauce, blend 4 dessert spoons of tahini, a big squeeze of lemon, a clove of garlic, some parsley and enough water to make yoghurt like consistency.

It is a bit messy so it is a good idea to make a big batch and freeze them and it is so cheap!

SPC Mousakka

(by Nawal Hassanyeh – Lovely Laura's Mum)

What can I say about Nawal?! Mother, chef, and the kindest woman in the universe... seriously. She is a great beautician and gives me the biggest, longest hugs in the world. Fabulous person.

Ingredients

- 2 aubergines;
- 2 large onions (slice each onion in 1/2 then slice 1 cm apart);
- 3 garlic cloves (each one sliced 4 times);
- 1 small can of chickpeas;
- 1 can chopped tomatoes;
- 2 bell peppers (red ones then choose between green or yellow – each one sliced 1 cm apart);
- 2 tablespoons tomato puree;
- Vegetable oil;

Method

Use a large pot to cook in.

Peel the aubergines but leave a couple of strips of the skin showing on them! Chop the aubergines in the middle then slice them a cm apart (make sure they are not thin).

Then use a frying pan with 3–4 tablespoons of oil – heat the oil well first before adding the aubergines to the pan.

Add about 4 at a time and fry both sides!! Make sure you do not burn them! The colour of them should be brown.

When you take them out of the pan, place them in a sieve on a plate to drain the excess oil and leave to one side. Heat pot with 1 tablespoon of vegetable oil, medium heat, and then add the onions and garlic. Stir from time to time, with the use of a wooden spoon, to prevent overcooking. When onions and garlic are much softer, add the chickpeas and use the wooden spoon to mix them with the onions by moving them from side to side, rather than stirring. Add the chopped tomatoes and bell peppers and repeat the same as you did with the chickpeas. Add seasoning such as sea salt, cinnamon, black and white pepper. At this point, add 1/2 mug of hot water to mix and make sauce. When it starts to boil a little, add 1 1/2 tablespoons of tomato puree in a separate bowl with 2 tablespoons of hot water and stir until the puree has fully melted, then add to the pot. Leave to cook for 5 minutes. Taste sauce and add seasoning to your own taste if you need to.

Switch on oven to 200°C. Get a Pyrex glass dish, and then use a large spoon with holes, and take out only the ingredients, leaving the sauce in the pot, and set the ingredients in the Pyrex. Then take the aubergines and place them neatly over the ingredients to cover them. Leave the sauce to cook and thicken slightly, but still allow being a bit runny in the pot (about 5 minutes). Then pour over the ingredients equally! Only apply the amount you need! Do not let dish overflow. Cover with foil and put in oven to cook for 30 minutes, then remove foil, turn down oven to 170°C, and leave to cook for 10–15 minutes. Keep an eye on it so it does not overcook. Take out of oven, leave to cool and then **ENJOY!!!**

This dish can be eaten hot and cold depending on your choice. You can also add chilli to it if you like.

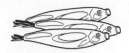

Smoked fish wraps

I cobbled this together one afternoon when I was craving paté and crisp bread. I love the soft mousse-like filling and the crunchy lettuce surround.

Ingredients

2 smoked mackerel fillets (I got them on offer in Tesco's);

1 small tin of tuna in oil (drain most of it off);

200g/4oz cottage cheese;

1 tablespoon organic cream or 1 teaspoon coconut oil;

Juice of half a lemon;

Pinch smoked paprika (or more to taste);

Freshly ground black pepper;

Pinch cayenne pepper;

Chopped parsley (optional);

Drained haricot beans.

Method

Tip the whole lot into a food processor. Blitz until mixed and smooth.

Serve in lettuce or chicory 'boats' – take one leaf of crisp iceberg lettuce or chicory and spoon some mixture into it, put a dessert spoon of haricot beans on top.

Roll the edges in (like a wrap) and eat away to your heart's content.

Perfect Chick snack – protein, pulses, vegetables.

Make a whole pot of it and store in the fridge! Can also be used as a good starter for dinner parties.

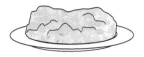

Haricot Mash

*A staple – it goes with **EVERYTHING!***

Take 1 or 2 tins of haricot beans in water (1 tin will give enough mash for two people). Drain them and rinse in lots of cold water. Put them in a saucepan with a glug of olive or macadamia nut oil. Warm them up slowly until the beans are warmed through.

Now comes the fun bit...

Add what ever herb spice combinations that you like.

Suggestions:
- Roasted garlic and chopped parsley;
- Smoked paprika;
- Cumin and cayenne;
- Unsweetened chilli sauce.

Yum x

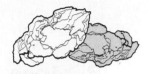

Onion Bhajis

OK Chicks...these things are like nuts...tough to eat only a few. They are a party treat really. The secret of these is to make only a small batch because they do not keep and so only make them when someone will share them with you. I suggest halving all these quantities. I do this so I do not choke down all 12 of the bhajis these quantities will make. Gram flour is made from a small chickpea so perfect for Six Pack Chicks. You can buy it in all large supermarkets.

Ingredients

(A deep saucepan and frying basket or a deep fat fryer is required.)

100g / 4oz gram flour;
1/4 teaspoon chilli powder;
1/2 teaspoon turmeric;
1/2 teaspoon baking powder;
Salt;

1/2 teaspoon ground cumin;
Large onion, halved and thinly sliced;
1 green chilli, deseeded and finely chopped;
25g / 1oz finely chopped

fresh coriander;
Cold water to mix;
Sunflower or groundnut oil for deep frying;

Method

Sift the flour, chilli, turmeric, cumin, baking powder and salt into a large mixing bowl.

Add the chopped coriander, onions and chillies and mix well.

Put on the extractor fan and open the windows – just to piss off the neighbours.

Preheat the deep fat fryer to 180°C / 350°F or the oil in a

saucepan.

Gradually add enough water to the flour mixture to form a thick batter mixing very well so the onions are well coated.

Very carefully, drop spoonfuls of the mixture into the hot oil and fry, and keep warm whilst you cook the remaining bhajis.

Drain well on kitchen paper and serve very hot.

Pinto Bean Dip

Perfect snacking food for chicks.

Ingredients

1 (15 oz) can pinto beans in water, rinsed and drained;

1/2 red pepper, finely chopped;

1 stalk celery, finely chopped;

1 small onion, finely chopped;

2 garlic cloves, minced;

2 teaspoons balsamic vinegar;

2 teaspoons lemon juice, freshly squeezed;

1 teaspoon dried oregano;

1/2 teaspoon ground cumin;

1/2 teaspoon smoked paprika (optional);

Ground black pepper;

2 pinches of sea salt (don't use table salt).

Method

You can use any beans for this recipe – borlotti beans work really well, too, if using them, then substitute dried basil for the cumin.

Drain beans in a sieve and rinse for 1 minute in running cold water. Throw everything into a food processor and blitz until smooth.

Try making different varieties – add any herbs or spices that you like!

Eat with raw veggies, preferably celery, peppers, cauliflower. Carrots are fine but don't overdo them – they are vegetable crack cocaine.

Delicious!

Chickpea, Aubergine and Tamarind Curry

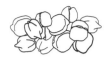

Ingredients

1 large aubergine;
Coconut oil;
1 large onion;
1 tablespoon finely chopped ginger;
1 tablespoon crushed garlic;
3 teaspoon garam masala;

1 teaspoon black mustard seeds;
1/2 pack tamarind paste (I used Seasoned Pioneers' 45g pouch and used the whole thing so I had to dilute the ingredients with a litre of water,

which also works really well);
1 large tin of chickpeas;
1 large courgette;
1 green pepper;
3–4 chilli peppers (potency of chilli is up to you!).

Method

Chop aubergine, courgette and green pepper into large chunks and massage in 1 tablespoon of coconut oil. Roast at 225°C in the oven for about 20 minutes until nicely browned. Chop onion and fry with the ginger and garlic in 1 tablespoon of coconut oil and when browning nicely, add the mustard seeds until the smell hits you. Then add the garam masala and cook for about 1 minute on a low-medium heat so as not to burn the spices. Add the tamarind paste and 500ml–700ml water and chopped chillies, and then boil. Turn down to a simmer and reduce slightly for about 5 minutes. When the vegetables are roasted, add to the pan with the chickpeas and sauce and season if needed. The tamarind gives a great flavour and so salt is not necessary. Eat with some grilled chicken and/or brown rice on 'kick ass' day (cheat day).

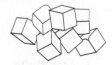

Vegetarian Tofu Scramble

(This recipe comes courtesy of Kip Dorrell –
www.messyvegetariancook.com)

*I met Kip years ago and her vegetarian/vegan recipes are superb. You can
enjoy this tofu scramble at any time of the day but I love it at breakfast.*

Ingredients

1 tablespoon water
(15ml);

¼ teaspoon black salt;

1/8 teaspoon turmeric;

2 cloves garlic, minced;

1 teaspoon coconut/
vegetable oil;

35g broccoli, cut into
small florets;

10–15g cashews, whole
or in pieces;

150g pressed firm tofu;

25g shredded kale;

1 small tomato (or

3–4 cherry sized
tomatoes), diced;

2 small spring onions,
white and green
parts, diced;

1–2 tablespoon
nutritional yeast.

Method

Mix the water, black salt,
turmeric, and garlic in a small
container and set aside.

Heat the oil in a wok or frying
pan to medium heat.

Add the broccoli and cashews;
stir frying for about a minute,
until the cashews develop some

brown spots.

Crumble the tofu into the pan
(there will be uneven sized lumps,
but you can break up any that
are too big with your cooking
implement).

Tip the kale in as well and stir-fry
for 3–4 minutes.

The tofu colour will change slightly, browning to a pale yellow.

Add the diced tomato and spring onions, stirring to mix through the scramble.

Pour the ingredients from step one into the pan and quickly stir to combine. Continue to stir moderately and after a minute sprinkle the nutritional yeast over the contents of the pan to soak up any remaining liquid.

To brown the scramble off, turn the heat up to high and rapidly stir-fry for another minute or two.

Serve over toast with your favourite sides and sauce. Vegetarian Worcestershire, Sri Racha, soy sauce (or tamari for gluten free) are some personal favourites.

The Protein Power Shake

Ingredients

1 scoop of your favourite protein powder;

Large glass of ice-cold water;

1 teaspoon of flaxseed powder;

1 teaspoon of macadamia nut oil;

Method

Throw all ingredients into a blender and blitz until smooth.

Use as a breakfast replacement or mid afternoon if you are exercising before you will get to eat dinner.

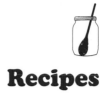

Recipes

Easy-peasy mayonnaise

Ingredients

2 free-range egg yolks (try and use Burford Browns);

1 free-range whole egg;

1 tablespoon French mustard;

½ lemon just the juice!

400ml/14¼fl oz

groundnut oil;

Salt and freshly ground black pepper;

Method

Throw all of the ingredients except the oil in a food processor and mix for 10–15 seconds, or until well combined. Then while the motor is running, pour the oil into the food processor very slowly until well combined and the mixture is thick and glossy. Finally, season to taste, with salt and freshly ground black pepper.

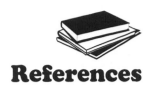

References

1. Marsh KA, et al. Effect of a low Glycaemic Index compared with a conventional healthy diet on polycystic ovary syndrome Am J Clin Nutr 19 May 2010.

2. Warburg O. On the origin of cancer cells. Science 1956 Feb; 123:309-14.

3. Volk T, et al. pH in human tumor xenografts: Effect of intravenous administration of glucose. Br J Cancer 1993 Sep; 68(3):492-500.

4. Digirolamo M. Diet and cancer: markers, prevention and treatment. New York: Plenum Press; 1994. p 203.

5. Leeper DB, et al. Effect of IV glucose versus combined IV. plus oral glucose on human tumor extracellular pH for potential sensitization to thermoradiotherapy. Int J Hyperthermia 1998 May–June; 14(3):257-69.

6. Rossi-Fanelli F, et al. Abnormal substrate metabolism and nutritional strategies in cancer management. JPEN J Parenter Enteral Nutr 1991 Nov–Dec; 15(6):680-3.

7. Grant JP. Proper use and recognised role of TPN in the cancer patient. Nutrition 1990 Jul–Aug; 6(4 Suppl):6S-7S, 10S.

8. American College of Physicians. Parenteral

nutrition in patients receiving cancer chemotherapy. Ann Intern Med 1989 May; 110(9):734.

9. Brand-Miller J, et al. The glucose revolution. Newport (RI) Marlowe and Co.; 1999.

10. Mooradian AD, et al. Glucotoxicity: potential mechanisms. Clin Geriatr Med 1999 May; 15(2):255.

11. Hoehn, SK, et al. Complex versus simple carbohydrates and mammary tumors in mice. Nutr Cancer 1979; 1(3):27.

12. Santisteban GA, et al. Glycaemic modulation of tumor tolerance in a mouse model of breast cancer. Biochem Biophys Res Commun 1985 Nov 15; 132(3):1174-9.

13. Seeley S. Diet and breast cancer: the possible connection with sugar consumption. Med Hypotheses 1983 Jul;11(3):319-27.

14. Sanchez A, et al. Role of sugars in human neutrophilic phagocytosis. Am J Clin Nutr 1973 Nov;26(11):1180-4.

15. Moerman CJ, et al. Dietary sugar intake in the aetiology of biliary tract cancer. Int J Epidemiol 1993 Apr;22(2):207-14.

16. Gatenby RA. Potential role of FDG-PET imaging in understanding tumor-host interaction. J Nucl Med 1995 May;36(5):893-9.

About the author

Bridget Hunt is the leader of the Six Pack Chick Company and 'Mother Hen' to all the clients in the dietary Facebook support group.

Bridget is a trained dancer and became interested in nutrition at the age of eighteen. Suffering from kidney problems, she set about improving her health and wellbeing by meeting Breda Gasjek from the British College of Nutrition and Health and going on to study.

Over the years, many fellow dancers and friends asked for her advice on nutrition, and how she trained her body to become stronger, fitter and healthier. Bridget studied Anatomy and Physiology and decided to train in Personal and Functional Training to assist her clients in overcoming injury – taking influence from an industry great, John Hardy, she trains clients to get the maximum out of every session leaving them feeling energised, balanced and confident.

Curious about how important a role the mind plays in weight loss, training and confidence, Bridget trained in NLP techniques to ensure clients not only lose the weight, but also keep it off. Her one-to-one sessions really do cover all aspects, ensuring an individual is left in control of what they eat and super confident in the way they look and feel.

Bridget gives talks to large groups on emotional eating, extreme fat loss and becoming a happier and slimmer version of **YOU**.

Bridget Hunt represents a role model to 1000s of women wanting to change, committing to change and who go on to help and influence others.

For more information contact:

www.sixpackchick.com

Motherhen@sixpackchick.com

www.facebook.com/sixpackchick

www.twitter.com/sixpackchick

Printed in Great Britain
by Amazon.co.uk, Ltd.,
Marston Gate.